HEALTH CONTINUUM AND DATA EXCHANGE IN BELGIUM AND IN THE NETHERLANDS

Studies in Health Technology and Informatics

This book series was started in 1990 to promote research conducted under the auspices of the EC programmes Advanced Informatics in Medicine (AIM) and Biomedical and Health Research (BHR), bioengineering branch. A driving aspect of international health informatics is that telecommunication technology, rehabilitative technology, intelligent home technology and many other components are moving together and form one integrated world of information and communication media.

The complete series has been accepted in Medline. In the future, the SHTI series will be available online.

Volume 110

Recently published in this series

Vol. 109. E.J.S. Hovenga and J. Mantas (Eds.), Global Health Informatics Education
Vol. 108. A. Lymberis and D. de Rossi (Eds.), Wearable eHealth Systems for Personalised Health Management – State of the Art and Future Challenges
Vol. 107. M. Fieschi, E. Coiera and Y.-C.J. Li (Eds.), MEDINFO 2004 – Proceedings of the 11th World Congress on Medical Informatics
Vol. 106. G. Demiris (Ed.), e-Health: Current Status and Future Trends
Vol. 105. M. Duplaga, K. Zieliński and D. Ingram (Eds.), Transformation of Healthcare with Information Technologies
Vol. 104. R. Latifi (Ed.), Establishing Telemedicine in Developing Countries: From Inception to Implementation
Vol. 103. L. Bos, S. Laxminarayan and A. Marsh (Eds.), Medical and Care Compunetics 1
Vol. 102. D.M. Pisanelli (Ed.), Ontologies in Medicine
Vol. 101. K. Kaiser, S. Miksch and S.W. Tu (Eds.), Computer-based Support for Clinical Guidelines and Protocols – Proceedings of the Symposium on Computerized Guidelines and Protocols (CGP 2004)
Vol. 100. I. Iakovidis, P. Wilson and J.C. Healy (Eds.), E-Health – Current Situation and Examples of Implemented and Beneficial E-Health Applications
Vol. 99. G. Riva, C. Botella, P. Légeron and G. Optale (Eds.), Cybertherapy – Internet and Virtual Reality as Assessment and Rehabilitation Tools for Clinical Psychology and Neuroscience
Vol. 98. J.D. Westwood, R.S. Haluck, H.M. Hoffman, G.T. Mogel, R. Phillips and R.A. Robb (Eds.), Medicine Meets Virtual Reality 12 – Building a Better You: The Next Tools for Medical Education, Diagnosis, and Care
Vol. 97. M. Nerlich and U. Schaechinger (Eds.), Integration of Health Telematics into Medical Practice
Vol. 96. B. Blobel and P. Pharow (Eds.), Advanced Health Telematics and Telemedicine – The Magdeburg Expert Summit Textbook

ISSN 0926-9630

Health Continuum and Data Exchange in Belgium and in the Netherlands

Proceedings of Medical Informatics Congress (MIC 2004) & 5th Belgian e-Health Conference

Edited by

Francis H. Roger France

Université Catholique de Louvain, Brussels, Belgium

Etienne De Clercq

Université Catholique de Louvain, Brussels, Belgium

Georges De Moor

Universiteit Gent, Ghent, Belgium

Johan van der Lei

Erasmus, MC, Universiteit van Rotterdam, Rotterdam, The Netherlands

IOS Press

Amsterdam • Berlin • Oxford • Tokyo • Washington, DC

ISBN 1 58603 487 1
Library of Congress Control Number: 2004115605

Publisher
IOS Press
Nieuwe Hemweg 6B
1013 BG Amsterdam
The Netherlands
fax: +31 20 620 3419
e-mail: order@iospress.nl

Distributor in the UK and Ireland
IOS Press/Lavis Marketing
73 Lime Walk
Headington
Oxford OX3 7AD
England
fax: +44 1865 750079

Distributor in the USA and Canada
IOS Press, Inc.
4502 Rachael Manor Drive
Fairfax, VA 22032
USA
fax: +1 703 323 3668
e-mail: iosbooks@iospress.com

PRINTED IN THE NETHERLANDS

Foreword

This book is the second to appear in the IOS Press "Studies in Health Technology and Informatics" in order to describe a follow up of research projects and the development of standards for "e-Health in Belgium and in the Netherlands".*

It is first based on the Belgo-Dutch Medical Informatics Congress **(Medische Informatica Congres), MIC 04**. Its Proceedings are published in the first part of this book. MICs started in Rotterdam, the Netherlands, in 1978 and in Antwerp in 1979, in Belgium. For its 22nd edition, it is held in Brussels on 25-26 November 2004.

The collection of papers covers timely areas such as nursing and care process, the electronic patient record and knowledge bases, as well as ICT assessment. Applications are described by short abstracts.

The second part of the book is devoted to the description of the development of standards by the Belgian Commission "Norms for Telematics in the Health Care Sector". It is a written support to the **"Telematics@health.be 5th Symposium"** held jointly with MIC04 in Brussels. A general introduction to the work of this Federal Commission in Belgium has been published in 2002.°

These two Conferences share new trends in health informatics and present many timely ideas and practical proposals. They are directed to health care professionals who are leading the transformation of health care by using information and knowledge.

MIC04 is organised by the two national societies for Medical Informatics : MIM (Medische Informatica, Informatique Médicale) in Belgium and VMBI (Vereniging voor informatie verwerking in de zorg) in the Netherlands.

Telematics@health.be is an annual symposium managed by the Public Federal Service of Public Health.

We wish to thank all authors, as well as reviewers of the papers, and translators of recommendations. We express also our gratitude to Mrs Chris De Hollander and Mrs Dominique Pironet for the follow up and the technical editing, as well as of Mrs Dominique Dieng from INFOPOLE for her support.

F.H. Roger France
E. De Clercq
G. De Moor
J. van der Lei

Editors

* F.H. Roger France, A. Hasman, E. De Clercq, G. De Moor
E-Health in Belgium and in the Netherlands, IOS Press, 2002, 93

° F.H. Roger France and M. Bangels
Norms for Telematics in Health Care : Priorities in Belgium
(in E-Health in Belgium and in the Netherlands, IOS 2002, 93, 179-183)

Contents

Application Session (Abstracts)

Part Two: Be-Health Related Topics

The Added Value of a Process Oriented Hospital Information System Supporting the Integrated Patient Care

Ilse LIESMONS
Administratief Centrum Caritas vzw,
Interleuvenlaan 10, 3001 Heverlee, Belgium
iliesmons@accnet.be

Abstract. This paper will demonstrate the added value of a Process Oriented Hospital Information System based on the current trends and changes in the organisation of patient care in hospitals. To support the integrated patient care with IT, basic functionalities will be described.

Keywords. Process Oriented Hospital Information System, Integrated electronic patient organizer, Clinical pathway, Computerized, Order communication

Introduction

The first part of this paper will be dedicated to the current developments in the organisation of patient care in hospitals, linked to the importance of a process oriented hospital information system. In the second part the consequences of an implementation process on the hospital structure will be analysed. Finally the basic functionalities necessary for an optimal process oriented hospital information system will be described.

1. Important Developments in the Organisation of Patient Care and the Effects on the ICT Components of a Modern Hospital Information System

1.1. Increasing Operational Care Efficiency

There is currently a clear trend in patient care towards increasing the productivity and controlling the cost. Each national government is confronted with the need to implement a health care policy that decreases the ever-raising expenses. On the other hand the population's need for care is increasing.

This situation where the care request (and the expenses linked to it) is increasing more rapidly than the government financing, leads to:

- an increase of private financing: the patient will have to pay more "out of pocket" resulting in a growing private insurance market.
- an ever-increasing pressure on hospital management to control its budget: to increase productivity and cost-effectiveness [9].

The pressure to increase the operational efficiency within the hospitals can be felt not only in the supporting processes but also in the basic care process. This pressure on the care process will continue in the future. Under government pressure the hospital basic care process has been influenced towards reducing the number of hospital days. Working with Diagnostic Rated Groups is the future: in Germany the new DRG system started on January 1, 2004. The government pays hospitals a fixed rate for each diagnosis regardless of how many days a patient stays in the hospital or the degree of costs incurred during that stay. This will cause a paradigm shift: the length of stay will no longer generate revenue; it will become the most important cost driver. In the future process management will be the keyword, in other words guiding the patient throughout the chain of tests and treatments. This creates an important additional requirement for the hospital information system: computerizing the patient care process and the expenses linked to it.

1.2. The Transition from Traditional Mono-Disciplinary Care to Multi-Disciplinary Care

The transition from traditional mono-disciplinary care to multi-disciplinary care has become an important issue for hospitals. Due to growing scientific knowledge and new medical technologies the care has become so complex and diversified that it has become impossible for one person to manage the clinical problem. A multi-disciplinary and multi-professional approach implies the cooperation of several medical and non-medical experts in the patient care process. Patient care is developing to an integrated, continuous, all inclusive care package bundling all professional health workers skills, each of them contributing his/her own specific expertise [6]. This represents a double challenge for the modern hospital information system. On the one hand there is the need to support the professionals to perform at their best in their indispensable individual professional expertise. On the other hand it must support a coherent team contributing to the complete patient care process.

1.3. Patient Care Intensification

An evolution is going on in the hospital treatment and care activity. Hospitals are changing into high-technology intervention centres. New diagnostic techniques lead to faster and more accurate patient care. New therapeutic technologies lead to a less invading, less aggressive and a more agreeable health care. Through these technological developments, hospitals are becoming specialized care institutions. This is the logical effect of a strong diagnostic and therapeutic process concentrated in an ever-shorting hospital stay. New information and communication technology makes it possible to bring the right patient information to the medical and nursing staff on an integrated way.

And exactly this point is important: the more intensive the care, the more frequent and nearer to the patient decisions need to be taken. It is a great advantage for the hospitals that the current information and communication technology allows an information decentralisation on an integrated way. The era of "island automation" and the result information fragmentation is definitely over [6].

1.4. The Patient Health Care Request is the Leading Factor

At this moment the nature and the amount of care given within hospitals is based on the care package, which is more or less "available" in the hospitals. Currently many of the diagnostic and therapeutic procedures and interventions are performed out of habit or for financial reasons, not necessarily what the patient requires. Times are changing. Home care, meaning that part of care, which takes part outside the hospital walls, is on its way up. It is obvious that in the future it will be necessary to have an information system, which sustains in a computerized way the extra-murus cooperation with the first line health caretaker.

In short: do whatever is necessary for the patient, do what connects to the specific care need, the patient care request and the patient's expectations, not less, not more but what is necessary. At this time a number of instruments are available to achieve this. These instruments have their relevant justification in common applying the principles of "evidence based clinical care": clinical practice codes, clinical pathways, evaluation protocols... These instruments have been invented for care processes and they enable to define the start of the care program [5].

2. The Effects on the Hospital Being an Organisation

2.1. The Functional Hospital Organisation

Hospitals often have a functional organisation structure based on input, more specifically using human resources, in general ordered on a functional department base: medical, nursing, administrative, technical, etc... Within the hospital these departments are usually structured in a hierarchical way.

Traditionally hospitals separate the clinical process from the management process. The board in a functional hospital organisation consists of a general director and the heads of the departments. The board is responsible for lining out the policy and executing the day to day hospital policy. The medical department represents the medical specialists. In first instance physicians are the clinical process managers.

Typical for these hospital organisations is that the physician and the operational units communicate using channels of medical prescription. This is no longer efficient.

An analysis of the activities of this kind of hospitals shows that only 24% of the time is dedicated to the basic hospital function: patient care and stay. 76% of the total time is dedicated to documentation, coordination, transport, supervision and waiting.

As we know from Abersnagel and Van Vliet [1], the Academic Hospital Utrecht, during an average process of a hospitalisation, meaning an eight to ten days stay, a patient goes through five departments, eighteen disciplines and meets more or less a hundred employees. The management process and the clinical process in this functional organisation communicate by a number of requests and prescriptions resulting in an overload of administration and communication. The different services treat all requests separately as if they were not connected.

When the hospital as well as the individual physicians try to achieve separately their proper efficiency without inter-tuning, it very often results into a mutual lack of understanding resulting in patient care deficiencies. A preliminary study of Vincent et al. [7] shows that from the 1 014 stays in two emergency hospitals of the Big-London area, in 10.8% of the cases unexpected events have happened of which 6% result in a permanent injury and 8% in a lethal ending.

2.2. A Process Guided Hospital Model

In a process guided hospital the patient is the basis for structuring the hospital organisation. The hospital process is the central axis shaping the care process.

According to Sermeus and Vleugels [6] by supporting the clinical process it will become possible to define the care concept in a better way, to respond in a better way to the patient needs and expectations, to enhance interdisciplinary and interprofessional coopera-

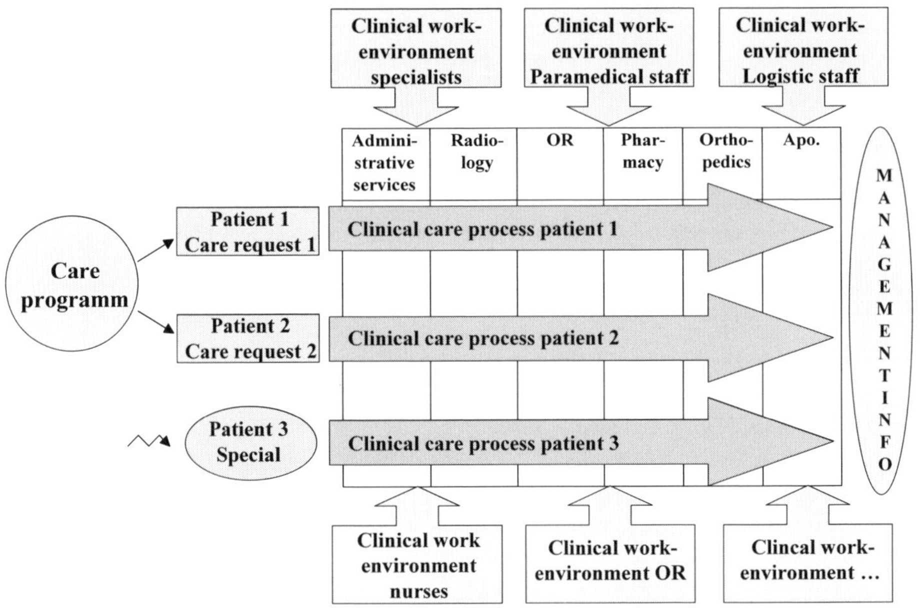

Figure 1. The patient, the central figure in the process oriented hospital information system. The patient will be assigned with his/her care request to a care program and will follow a specific care process. In exceptional cases the patients will be assigned to a individual treatment plan.

tion. Clinical care quality criteria and objectives can be established. This way a full program in the shape of a care program can be offered to the patient instead of a series of separated, uncoordinated interventions.

Hospitals that have instituted clinical pathways have seen substantial improvements in both clinical and operational dimensions. Efficiency in clinical operations requires administrators to manage three things well: patient throughput (getting the right patient in the right bed at the right time), clinical resource management (using the right supplies, drugs and devices), and nursing (delivering the appropriate treatment team at all times) [4].

By introducing clinical pathways in the United States, length of stay has fallen by 33 %. Hospitals that have instituted clinical pathways have seen substantial improvement in both clinical and operational dimensions. In one specific hospital the introduction of clinical pathways brought about 25% reduction in average length of stay across the hospital, which reduced overall costs by approximately 10% [2].

3. The Process Guided Hospital Information System

In the above sections we have tried to show the importance of a process-oriented hospital. To support this process with IT we will establish in the following sections the basic functionalities necessary for **an operational process oriented hospital information system.** A reference site where the integrated system is up and running is the Maaslandziekenhuis Sittard-Netherlands. In Germany round 130 hospitals are working on the process oriented way. A few examples are Charité Universitätsmedizin Berlin Campus Benjamin Franklin (1255 beds); Klinikum der Friedrich-Schiller-Universität Jena (1394 beds); Klinikum der Universität Regensburg (804 beds); Krankenhaus Bad soden (327 beds).[3]

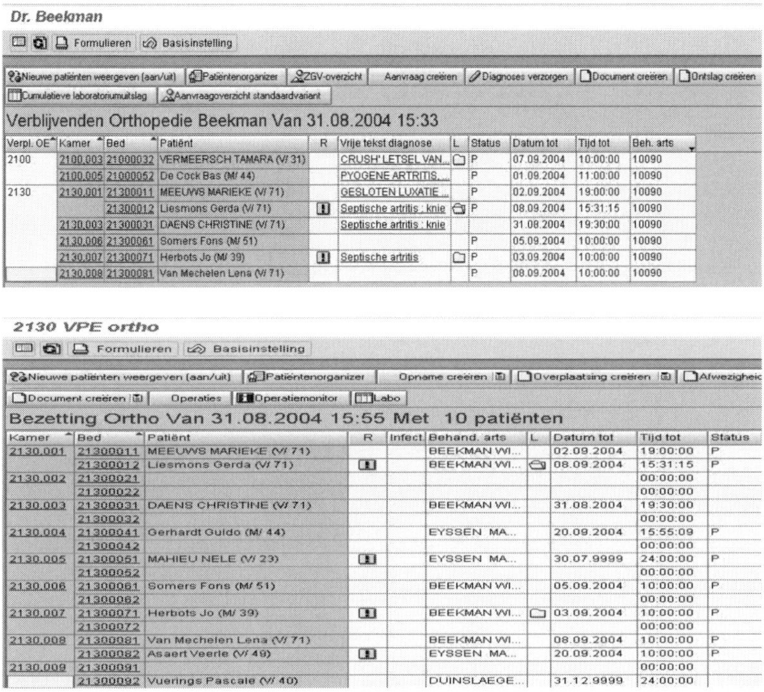

Figure 2. A clinical work environment gives the multi-disciplinary team members an optimal follow-up of the patient care process and results in big administrative simplification.

3.1. Electronic Work Environment for all Multidisciplinary Team Members

Once the patient is assigned to a specific care program by the physician, the patients individual care process can start. The patient will go through a number of hospital services, each of them administering a part of the care, during which he/she will meet different care professionals who are member of a multidisciplinary team. Each team member will contribute to the care program from his/her own clinical work environment. Each team member will have his own personalised view on the patient. The sample screens below give a view of a clinical work environment of a physician and a nurse of the patients on the a working day. The physician has a view on his own hospitalised patients while the nurse on the other hand has a view of all hospitalised patients on the ward she is working on. Both displays are integrating the same data, which are entered only once in the central database. From this view specialists and nurses have the possibility to consult lab results, RX protocols, anamneses documents,…

3.2. Order Communication

The ability to electronically request orders by means of order communication is another important functionality. Starting from a central environment the physician can request all kinds of tests electronically, e.g. medical technical tests such as lab, RX, anatomic pathology or the opinion of another physician specialist, appointments, bed planning, electronic request for operation theatre-planning, etc….

At all times the physician has an overview of the orders he asked for a particular patient included an integrated overview of the results and protocols.

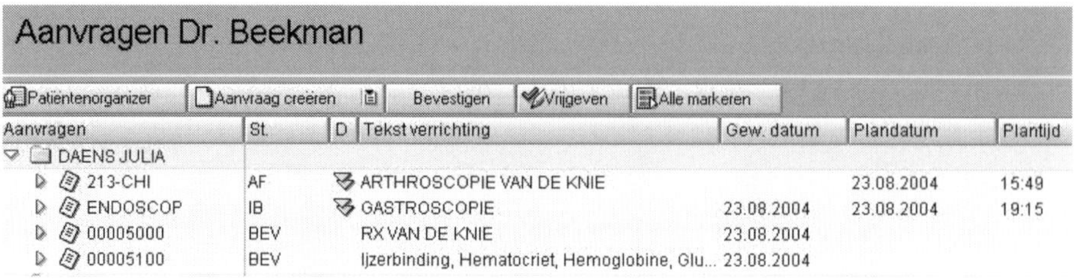

Figure 3. An overview of requested orders, results and protocols from the work environment of the physician.

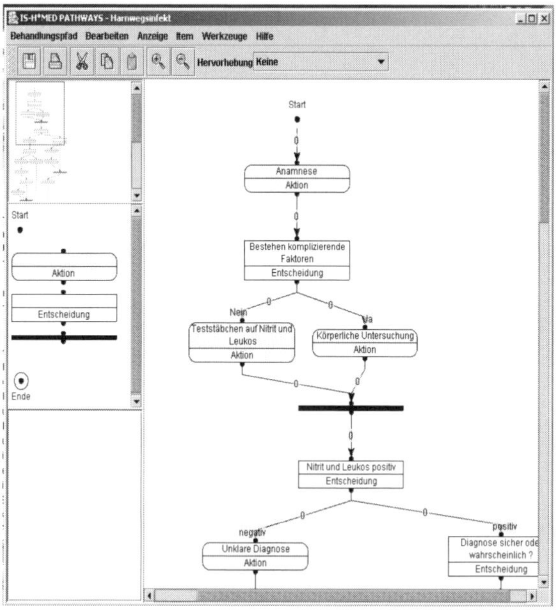

Figure 4. Computerised clinical pathway.

3.3. Patient Clinical Treatment Process

A clinical pathway is a method for organising the patient's care in the hospital intended to produce the best health outcome in the shortest time using the fewest resources. Patients are assigned to a specific pathway by their admitting diagnoses. The pathway includes a day-by-day checklist of the care the patient should receive, incorporating diagnostic tests, medical therapy, and other therapeutic interventions. The daily checklists permit hospitals more accurately to assess demand for services. Having a daily plan of care helps physicians align themselves with the patient's and hospital's best interests. It reminds the physician of best practices, helps them organize their day, reduces the amount of effort devoted to documentation, improves communication to nursing staff and all the other members of the multidisciplinary team, synchronizes expectations and underlines the importance of starting discharge planning at the time of admission [2]. As shown below, it is possible to call the patient clinical treatment pathway function from the clinical work station of the physician. In addition, it is possible to adjust the layout of the clinical work station so that it becomes clear whether pathways are assigned, whether tasks have to be completed…

The component contains the following tools for creating and using patient clinical treatment pathways:

Tool	Function
System Administration	Creation of new treatment pathways and changing existing pathways.
Monitor	Overview of all treatment pathways. Performances of the necessary activities, e.g. activate, deactivate, transport.
Patient Pathway Assignment	Assignment of predefined treatment pathways to patients. These then become patient pathways.
Patient Pathway Processing	Patient pathways are displayed as work lists. The user can process the individual steps, display relevant information, or trigger system activities.

Figure 5. Tools for creating and using patient clinical treatment pathways.

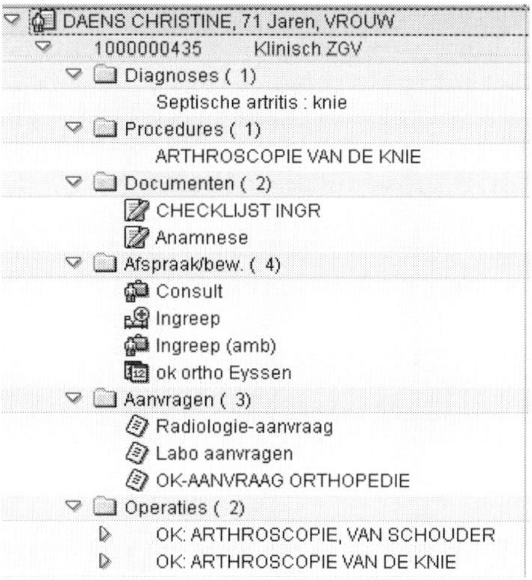

Figure 6. Patient organizer.

3.4. The Integrated Management of the Electronic Patient File Data in the Patient Organizer

The next important step in the integrated computerization of the patient care process is the central management of the electronic patient file. Through the electronic patient organizer the patient history, the anamnesis, the electronic order requests, the result, the medical documents, the diagnosis, master patient files, etc.... is available. All multidisciplinary team members will have access, from their own working environment, to the information which is/or will be relevant for them. Even more, the electronic patient organizer offers a central and structured survey of all patient linked data with the possibility to change this data a.o. to create, modify, consult, erase, search...[8]. The patient organizer gives a status of the patient data: medical history, the current status (requests and results, executed/viewed) and even gives the possibility to verify what has been planned on a later date.

3.5. The Electronic Patient Data Access

It will be possible for the general practitioner, other referring institutions, physical therapists, home nurses and other caretakers, who are involved in the patient care process, to access the electronic patient file data through the internet. The process oriented hospital information system makes networking possible, which will lead to better quality of the patient care.

4. Conclusion

Working with a process oriented hospital information system is the computerized answer to a number of modern developments within the health care. They are: the need of an increasing operational and financial care efficiency, the need of transparent policy information, the transit of mono-disciplinary care towards multi-disciplinary care, a support to increase patient care intensification, the trans-murus patient information availability,... A very important aspect in the response to these tendencies is the need for the hospitals themselves to evolve from a functional hospital organisation towards a process oriented hospital. Using the patient care request in the clinical paths will not only improve the clinical practice but also lead to the correct policy information. Hospital will be more transparent and efficient as decisions will be made on facts

In order to be able to evolve to a fully process oriented hospital system a process oriented hospital information system should be based on offering automated concepts such as: patient clinical care process, an electronic working environment setup for all multi-disciplinary team members, order communication between the operational departments, central data management through patient organizer and the electronic and extra-murus access the patient data.

References

[1] Abersnagel, E en Van Vliet, J., *De invulling van kwalificatieniveau* 5, TVZ, 17, pp. 506-507, 1998.

[2] Buescher B., Kocher B., Russell R., Wichels R., *Pathways to productivity.*, Mc Kinsey Health Europe, number 3, March, pp. 51-59, 2004.

[3] Gesellschaft für Systemforschung und Dienstleistugen im Gesundheitswesen : IS-H Med; *The solution for SAP in the Hospital,* 1-43, 2002.

[4] Kempeneers N., *Kostencalculatie via E.R.P.-oplossing, financiële performantie van zorgprogramma's: Het einde van het laken?* K.U. Leuven Permanente vorming, Centrum voor ziekenhuis- en verplegingswetenschap, 8 maart 2002.

[5] Sermeus, W., Vanhaecht, K. en Vleugels, A., The Belgian-Dutch clinical Pathway Network., *Journal of Integrated Care Pathways*, 5,1, pp. 10-14, 2001.

[6] Sermeus, W., Vleugels, A., *Patiëntgestuurde organisatie.*, Management in de gezondheidszorg, 2002.

[7] Vincent, C, Neale, G. en Woloshynowych, M., *Advers events in British hospitals: preliminary retrospective record review*, BMJ, 322, 7285, pp. 517-519, 2001.

[8] Von Olaf D., *Patientenorganizer: Die elektronischen Patientenakte in IS-H*Med Forum. Krankenhaus IT, Die Zeitschrift für alle IT-Verantwortlichen im gesundheitswesen.* Nr 4 pp. 30-31, 2003.

[9] Watson, R., *European countries face similar problems of demographic ageing and higher patient expectations*, Britisch Medical Journal, 15 december 2001, 323:1388. www.rcn.org.uk.

Classifying Clinical Pathways

Leentje DE BLESER, *MSc, RN* [a], Joan VLAYEN, *MD* [b],
Kris VANHAECHT, *MSc, RN* [a] and Walter SERMEUS, *PhD, RN* [a]
[a]*Centre for Health Services Research, Catholic University of Leuven, Leuven, Belgium*
[b]*Center for Evidence Based Medicine (CEBAM), Belgium*

Abstract. Background: Clinical pathways are commonly developed for homogenous patient groups. We were wondering if the traditional patient classification systems could be used for classifying clinical pathways.

Methodology: To examine the utility of patient classification systems for clinical pathways, a sample of 13 clinical pathways was analyzed, involving a total of 412 patients. Three classification systems were tested: International Classification of Diseases, Ninth Revision (ICD9-CM), Clinical Coding System (CCS) data and All-Patient Redefined Diagnosis Related Groups (APR-DRG).

Results: Categorization with ICD9-CM and CCS shows rather wide variation. However, when restricting for the principal codes, CCS classification shows an almost homogeneous relationship with clinical pathways. APR-DRG's are already corrected for secondary procedures and are difficult to assess. Categorization with the Risk Of Mortality (ROM) is more homogeneous than with the Severity Of Illness (SOI).

Conclusion: Patient groups in clinical pathways are rather heterogeneous. When restricting for the principal procedures, the strongest relationship seems to exist between clinical pathways and CCS. Further research is needed to refine this relationship.

Keywords. Clinical pathway, Diagnosis Related Groups, Classification

Introduction

Clinical pathways are defined as "Schedules of medical and nursing procedures, including diagnostic tests, medications, and consultations designed to effect an efficient, coordinated program of treatment" [2]. Clinical pathways have several goals: reduction of unintended variation in care delivery, patient education, reduction in resource utilization, and improvement in quality of care [5,9]. One of the characteristics of clinical pathways is that they are mainly developed for homogenous patient groups [4]. Generally, specific inclusion and exclusion criteria are used to decide if a patient is taken into a clinical pathway. Because of this characteristic, classification systems can be used to classify clinical pathways. Well-known examples of classification systems are the International Classification of Diseases, Ninth Revision, Clinical Modification (ICD9-CM), the Clinical Coding System (CCS) and the All-Patient Redefined Diagnosis Related Groups (APR-DRG).

International Classification of Diseases, Ninth Revision (ICD9-CM) is based on the ICD9 coding, that was developed to classify mortality data in a more consistent way.

However, the ICD9-CM also maps morbidity data and has a special section to code procedures. This coding system has approximately 12 000 different codes for diagnosis and 3500 codes for procedures [6]. A key-characteristic of ICD-9 is that it is classifying diagnoses and procedures and is not classifying patients. One patient can have more problems or procedures which lead to more than one code per patient.

Clinical Coding System (CCS) is a tool for grouping conditions and procedures into a manageable number of clinically meaningful categories (Agency for Healthcare Research and Quality (AHRQ) [1]. This 'clinical grouper' makes it easier to quickly understand patterns of diagnosis and procedures so that health plans, policymakers, and researchers can analyze costs, utilization, and outcomes associated with particular illnesses and procedures. CCS consists of two related classification systems, single level and multilevel CCS. Single level CCS is most useful for ranking diagnoses and procedures. Multi-level CCS is most useful when evaluating larger aggregations of conditions and procedures or exploring them in greater detail. Because CCS is only a clinical grouper of ICD-9 codes, there can be more than 1 code per patient.

Diagnosis Related Groups (DRG's) are systems for classifying patients by relating common characteristics such as diagnosis, treatment, and age to an expected consumption of hospital resources and length of stay. Its purpose is to provide a framework for specifying case mix and to reduce hospital costs and reimbursement. In fact, it is the cornerstone of the prospective payment system [3]. In this patient classification system, the major diagnosis (coded in ICD9-CM) is first categorized in one of the Major Diagnostic Categories (MDC) – a classification based on the organ systems. Each MDC is divided according to the presence or absence of a surgical intervention of technique that takes place in an operation room. The surgical and medical subgroups are further divided according to age, complications and associated disorders. In this way, the categorization is determined by two processes: the management and the clinical process [7]. There is only one DRG-group per patient. In the 15th version, All Patient Refined – Diagnosis Related Groups (APR-DRG's), 355 different groups are identified. These groups are subdivided in four groups according to severity-of-illness (SOI) or risk of mortality (ROM).

1. Methodology

Thirteen surgical clinical pathways were included in this study [8]. These pathways are part of a broader Belgian federal project evaluating the quality of clinical pathways for patients undergoing a surgical intervention (ref. Onderzoeksrapport). Hospitals participating in this project were asked to collect data of a representative sample of patients passing through a pathway. Inclusion in a clinical pathway was done prospectively by the multidisciplinary team. The data were collected between January 2002 and June 2003.

Retrospectively, this information was compared with data from the hospital discharge dataset that are collected compulsory in Belgian Hospital (Royal Decree of June, 21 1990). Based on the ICD-9-CM registration, CCS-codes and APR-DRG groups were derived based on their respectively AHRQ- and 3M-algorithms (http://www.hcup-us.ahrq.gov/toolssoftware/ccs/ccs.jsp).

2. Results

The study sample consisted of 13 surgical clinical pathways. In total, 412 patients were included in these clinical pathways, ranging from 7 to 112 patients per pathway. The clinical pathways were developed for a broad range of pathologies: total hip arthroplasty (2), total knee arthroplasty, Anterior Lumbar Intervertebral Fusion (ALIF), Anterior Cervical Intervertebral Fusion (ACIF), low back surgery, cataract surgery, intracranial tumors, maxillary surgery, radical prostatectomy, abdominal hysterectomy, mammary carcinoma and caesarean section (Table 1).

Table 1. Description of the sample of clinical pathways.

Clinical pathway	Hospital	Period data collection	N
Total hip arthroplasty	Hospital 1	01-06/2003	42
Total knee arthroplasty	Hospital 2	01-06/2003	37
Cataract	Hospital 3	01-06/2003	97
Mammary carcinoma	Hospital 4	01-06/2003	112
Total hip arthroplasty	Hospital 5	07-12/2002	7
ALIF	Hospital 5	07-12/2002	15
ACIF	Hospital 5	01-12/2002	15
Low back surgery	Hospital 5	01-06/2002	15
Intracranial tumors	Hospital 5	01-12/2002	15
Maxillary operation	Hospital 5	01-12/2002	16
Radical prostatectomy	Hospital 5	01-12/2002	11
Abdominal hysterectomy	Hospital 5	07-12/2002	15
Caesarean section	Hospital 5	01-12/2002	15

Table 2. Number of different ICD9-CM, CCS and APR-DRG codes per clinical pathway.

Clinical pathway	N	ICD9-CM	CCS	APR-DRG
Total hip arthroplasty	42	2	2	1
Total knee arthroplasty	37	22	13	1
Cataract	97	7	4	3
Mammary carcinoma	112	47	32	8
Total hip arthroplasty	7	3	3	1
ALIF	15	4	3	1
ACIF	15	2	2	1
Low back surgery	15	3	2	1
Intracranial tumors	15	7	7	1
Maxillary operation	16	12	8	1
Radical prostatectomy	11	9	9	1
Abdominal hysterectomy	15	17	14	3
Caesarean section	15	10	7	1

Table 3. Number of principal ICD9-CM and CCS codes.

Clinical pathway	N	ICD9-CM	CCS
Total hip arthroplasty	42	1	1
Total knee arthroplasty	37	2	1
Cataract	97	3	1
Mammary carcinoma	112	5	2
Total hip arthroplasty	7	1	1
ALIF	15	1	1
ACIF	15	1	1
Low back surgery	15	1	1
Intracranial tumors	15	1	1
Maxillary operation	16	2	1
Radical prostatectomy	11	1	1
Abdominal hysterectomy	15	1	1
Caesarean section	15	1	1

The number of different ICD9-CM codes for each clinical pathway varies from 2 to 47 (Table 2). There is also a strong variation in the total number of ICD9-CM codes per pathway. When the ICD9-CM data are categorized according to the CCS classification system, there is only slightly less variation (2 to 32 CCS categories per pathway). Classification

Table 4. Number of patients within each pathway classified according to the Severity Of Illness.

Clinical pathway	N	Categories Severity Of Illness			
		1	2	3	4
Total hip arthroplasty	42	23	17	1	1
Total knee prosthesis	37	27		9	1
Cataract	97	80	16	1	
Mammary carcinoma	112	59	52	1	
ALIF	15	12	3		
ACIF	15	12	3		
Low back surgery	15	13	2		
Intracranial tumors	15	2	1	11	1
Maxillary operation	16	16			
Radical prostatectomy	11	9	2		
Abdominal hysterectomy	15	8	7		
Caesarean section	15	8	6	1	
Total	412	276	109	24	3

Table 5. Number of patients within each pathway classified according to the Risk Of Mortality.

Clinical pathway	N	Categories Risk Of Mortality			
		1	2	3	4
Total hip arthroplasty	42	30	10	1	1
Total knee arthroplasty	37	36	1		
Cataract	97	94	3		
Mammary carcinoma	112	105	6	1	
Total hip arthroplasty	7	7			
ALIF	15	15			
ACIF	15	15			
Low back surgery	15	15			
Intracranial tumors	15	2	9	3	1
Maxillary operation	16	16			
Radical prostatectomy	11	9	2		
Abdominal hysterectomy	15	13		2	
Caesarean section	15	15			
Total	412	372	31	7	2

with APR-DRG's shows the least variation, with 1 to 8 APR-DRG's per clinical pathway (Table 2). Three of the 13 clinical pathways have more than one APR-DRG.

When restricting to the principal diagnoses (Table 3), there still exists some variation in the number of principal ICD9-CM codes. When the ICD9-CM data are categorized according to the CCS classification system, there are less categories than with the ICD9-CM system. In other words, different principal ICD9-CM diagnoses are categorized in the same CCS code. As an exception, for the clinical pathway 'mammary carcinoma' there still exist 2 CCS codes (mastectomy and tumorectomy). Also, in the Total Knee Arthroplasty clinical pathway, one patient had a revision of the knee, which explains the second code. APR-DRG's are already taking the secondary diagnoses into account into one DRG-group per patient.

Although most patients are categorized in SOI category 1 or 2 (93,4 %), still a considerable number of patients have a higher SOI category (6,6 %), again stressing the heterogeneity of the patient groups (Table 4). This variation is less clear for the ROM, with only few patients classified in ROM category 3 or 4 (2,1 %, Table 5). The analysis clearly shows that the clinical pathways are more oriented to the less severe, more predictable patient groups.

3. Discussion

In this study, the relationship of clinical pathways with three patient classification systems was explored. A wide variation of ICD9-CM codes per clinical pathway was found, with up to 47 different codes in one pathway. This variation can be explained by the variable number of additional diagnoses and procedures in each clinical pathway. Less but still considerable variation can be found when categorization is done with CCS, which is based on ICD9-CM. When we restrict the coding to the principal diagnosis or procedure and grouping the ICD9-CM-codes into the CCS classification, clinical pathways can be classified in an acceptable homogeneous way.

The relationship between clinical pathways and APR-DRG's is also very strong, although approximately one in four included clinical pathways had more than one APR-DRG. This can be explained by the presence of several co-morbidities related to the disorder or the existence of several treatment options (e.g. mammary carcinoma). In the ideal and most simple situation, patients included in a clinical pathway are categorized in one APR-DRG, e.g. in the case of radical prostatectomy. However, some APR-DRG's are the basis for different clinical pathways. APR-DRG 302 for example categorizes patients with total hip prosthesis and total knee prosthesis.

Important heterogeneity is found within a DRG, looking to differences in SOI. This can be explained by the fact that clinical pathways are prospective instruments. In contrast, APR-DRG's are retrospective instruments, giving the possibility to take complications into account. Categorization with the ROM gives more homogeneous results, but further research is needed to compare the accuracy of the ROM and the SOI.

An important limitation of the present study is the small number of patients included in some of the clinical pathways. Therefore, additional research with a larger sample of pathways and patients will be needed to refine these results.

4. Conclusion

A rather high heterogeneity was found in the patient groups included in the present study when categorization was done with ICD9-CM, CCS and SOI. More homogeneous results can be achieved with ROM and APR-DRG's. These results can also be achieved for CCS, when restricted for the principal procedure codes. However, this more homogeneous relationship between clinical pathways and CCS/APR-DRG's will have to be refined in larger studies.

Acknowledgment

The project about clinical pathways is supported and financed by the Belgian federal Ministry of Public Health, Safety of Food Chain and the Environment.

References

[1] Agency for Healthcare Research and Quality (AHRQ). Clinical Classificiation Software 2004. 1-16. 2004. Maryland, HCUP.
[2] Anderson, K. (2000). Mosby's Medical, Nursing & Allied Health Dictionary. (W B Saunders).
[3] Bardsley, M., Coles, J., and Jenkins, L. (1989). DRGs and Health Care: The management of case mix. (King Edward's Hospital Find for London: London.).

[4] Coffey, R. J., Richards, J. S., Remmert, C. S., LeRoy, S. S., Schoville, R. R., and Baldwin, P. J. (1992). An introduction to critical paths. *Qual. Manag. Health Care* **1**, 45-54.
[5] Glauber, J. H., Farber, H. J., and Homer, C. J. (2001). Asthma clinical pathways: toward what end? *Pediatrics* 107, 590-592.
[6] Practice Management Information Corporation (1998). International Classification of Diseases 9th Revision, clinical modification, fifth edition. (PMIC: California.).
[7] Sermeus, W. (2003). De Belgische ziekenhuisfinanciering ontcijferd. (Acco: Leuven.).
[8] Sermeus, W., Ramaekers, D., Aertgeerts, B., Demeulemeester, E., Vlayen, J., and De Bleser, L. Tussentijds BOS-rapport Klinische Paden. 1-245. 2004. Leuven, unpublished work.
[9] Vanhaecht, K, Sermeus, W., Vleugels, A., and Peeters, G. (2002). Ontwikkeling en gebruik van klinische paden (clinical pathways) in de gezondheidszorg. *Tijdschrift voor Geneeskunde* 58, 1542-1551.

Address for correspondence

Mrs. Leentje De Bleser
Centre for Health Services Research
Catholic University of Leuven
Kapucijnenvoer 35/4
B-3000 Leuven
Belgium
Phone: +32 16336971
Fax: +32 16336970
e-mail: Leentje.debleser@med.kuleuven.ac.be

Introduction of Wireless Integrated Care Plans at the Bedside

Tom FIERS, Dirk LEMAITRE and Christophe JOLIE
University hospital Gent, De Pintelaan 185, 9000 Gent

Abstract. For years electronic care plans have been touted as an important tool to provide better patient care. Until recently however, most efforts were hampered by design gaps in available Electronic Patient Record (EPR) systems and the difficulties involved in extending continuous care to the bedside. The growth in wireless LAN solutions, and the emerging maturity of EPR systems have finally made practical implementations possible. An extensive analysis, development and preparation phase followed by a pilot on the department of traumatology in the University hospital of Gent has proven the possibilities and validity of multidisciplinary electronic care plans as an integral part of the EPR. Wireless consultation, observation and charting enables bedside management of patient care. Roll-out on 5 more departments is planned in the coming year.

Keywords. Hospital Information Systems, Critical Pathways, Quality of Health Care, Patient Care Planning, Outcome Assessment, Local Area Networks, Radio Waves

Introduction

Recent years have seen a coming of age of EPR (Electronic Patient Record) developments in many hospitals, resulting in many cases in a gradual shift from merely result servers to an increased focus on integrated care, order-communication solutions and implementing clinical pathways by using care plans embedded within the EPR [1]. Widespread availability and growing popularity of wireless local area networks (WLANs) for the general public on the other hand have led to an increased interest from healthcare institutions into wireless solutions, a necessity to the provision of bedside care. Lack of these possibilities has in the past often limited potential benefits of ordercommunication and care planning [2, 3].

In the university hospital of Gent a pilot study to bring wireless clinical pathways to the bedside started in March 2004 on the department of traumatology by using portable computers attached to the nursing ward trolleys. It has been used as a test bank for the technology involved and as a validation centre for bedside integrated care management. Rollout in the hospital will proceed with two further full departments by the end of the year.

1. Setting up a WLAN

Wireless LAN's became mainstream with the release of the 802.11 standard by the IEEE [4] in 1999. The original standard was limited to 2Mbps however. 802.11a offered speeds up to 54Mbps, but uses the 5GHz spectrum and therefore has a very limited range and would require an unreasonable number of antennas for an institution. The real breakthrough came with the arrival of 802.11b, and more recently 802.11g, both utilizing the 2.4GHz spectrum resulting in increased range. Theoretically, a range of 100m or more is possible in open air. In 802.11b speeds up to 11Mbps could be achieved, for g this is for now a theoretical maximum of 54Mbps, with the promise of a tenfold increase in 802.11n.

However in a hospital environment 'open air' is a euphemism as concrete, steel beams, elevators, isolation chambers and heavy equipment all combine to limit achievable range and throughput dramatically. Typically for 802.11g, about 10m to about the first wall is achievable at full speed, but very rapidly transfer speeds degrade to 11Mbps or lower, resulting in the need for more antennas. For a typical hospital ward, 3-4 antennas are necessary to insure full bedside coverage. Therefore investing in hospital wide WLAN technology is quite a considerable investment, even not taking into account interference, roaming, security issues and organisation [5].

1.1. Data Over DECT

In our hospital as in many others DECT (Digital Enhanced Cordless Telecommunications) networks have been installed to handle telephony. A first pilot WLAN was set up to reutilize the existing DECT antenna network, by using dedicated PCMCIA-DECT cards in portable computers. On the plus side was the already installed network, the adequate range and a relative security bonus as the hardware needed for data over DECT networks is not mainstream. As the bandwidth of a data over DECT network is quite limited (from 32Kbps up to 2Mbps depending on DECT architecture), Clinical Workstation (the UZ Gent EPR client-server application) was set up to run in a Citrix [6] environment, so reasonable speed could be achieved.

Extensive testing on 8 beds during some months revealed quite some initial problems with connections and roaming (switching from one antenna to another). Changes in organisation and hardware were necessary to handle 24 hour uptime requirements (extra batteries, chargers, recharging procedures etc). Although most of the problems were solved, carefree roaming could not be guaranteed at all times, resulting in rare but very user-unfriendly connectivity problems. Also the limited bandwidth of data over DECT prohibits usage of graphic-extensive parts of the EPR such as a PACS client and would also limit future expansion possibilities.

1.2. 802.11b/g Based Network

Due to the experiences with DECT more recently attention focused on implementing an additional 802.11 based network in the hospital. The fairly limited range and need for multiple antennas for each nursing ward requires careful planning. In Europe 13 channels are available for 802.11b and g. As there is a lot of interference from one channel to another, antennas on a ward can only use channels fairly distant from one another (e.g. 1, 6 and 11). Interference from one floor to another also has to be taken into account as nursing wards are located on different floors. To solve this adjustable antenna strength is a necessity for the access points. Access points have to be non-routing, so that roaming is not a problem. Although available 802.11 WLAN technology has significantly improved over the last two years and is off the shelf technology, a number of issues remain with different vendors such as automatic roaming which is not always switching as fast as it should (e.g. keeping a 2 Mbps connection when the trolley is nearer an 54Mbs connection), access points which power down temporarily when no activity is measured, or wireless traffic problems with some applications. On the plus side, connectivity is sometimes slowed down but never lost and much higher average speeds can be guaranteed, eliminating the need for the Citrix solution and opening the door to graphic intensive applications.

1.3. Security

Security is a big issue with WLAN's, as the network is by nature more accessible than a wired LAN. Certainly in a hospital setting, wireless data protection is an important factor to consider [7, 8]. The standard WLAN WEP (wired equivalent privacy) security layer which encrypts messages with a static key known to access point and client can easily be broken in some hours, even if additional security measures such as hiding network identifications, channels and limiting access to known computers (MAC filtering) were taken [9]. Currently the best option is to implement WPA (Wi-Fi Protected Access), which utilizes some of the features of the new 802.11i standard. By using WPA each packet gets its own ever-changing encryption, and authentication is enforced using 802.1x and authentication servers, such as RADIUS (Remote Authentication Dial-In User Service). In our hospital an additional firewall has been installed between the WLAN and LAN in order to further minimize the potential risks.

2. Introduction of Bedside Integrated Care Plans

2.1. Design and Implementation

During the previous years, a lot of effort has gone into the rollout of the basic EPR functionalities in our hospital. Simultaneously, in order to further improve continuity and coordination of care, an evolution to clinical pathways was prepared since 2001, with the cooperation of all users involved, in order to achieve optimal results. Clinical pathways are structured, multidisplinary plans of care designed to support the implementation of clinical guidelines and protocols. All existing procedures were gathered and structured in order to create the order sets and standing orders needed for care plans. Observations, progress charting and outcome goals were defined. The classical nursing record thus forms a subset of a care plan. The EPR software was adapted in order to cater for these extended needs. Thus a typical care plan is presented as a collection of all planned activities for a patient, visualised over a given time span. Nursing orders, medical orders, paramedical orders, problems, goals, exception charting and observations all form an integral part of it. The medication module also forms part of the care plan but has been separately evaluated up to now and has not yet been activated in the production environment in order not to complicate the initial care plan pilot. Also, from literature, benefits of physician order entry for medication still seem doubtful [10, 11], so integration in the integrated care plans will proceed carefully.

Depending on the needs, medical pathology and complexity of each department, different standard multidisciplinary care plans and observation lists are predefined with their associated problems and outcomes.

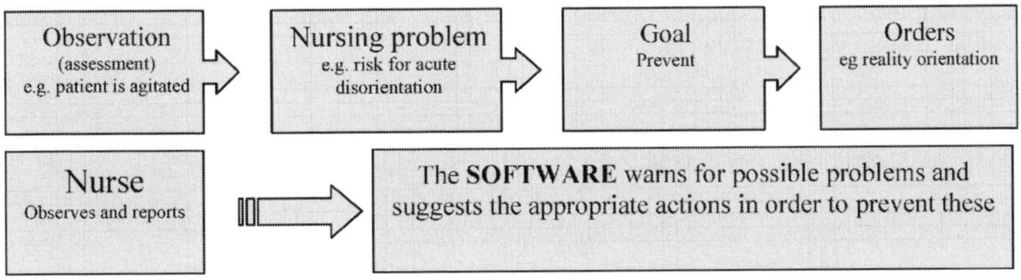

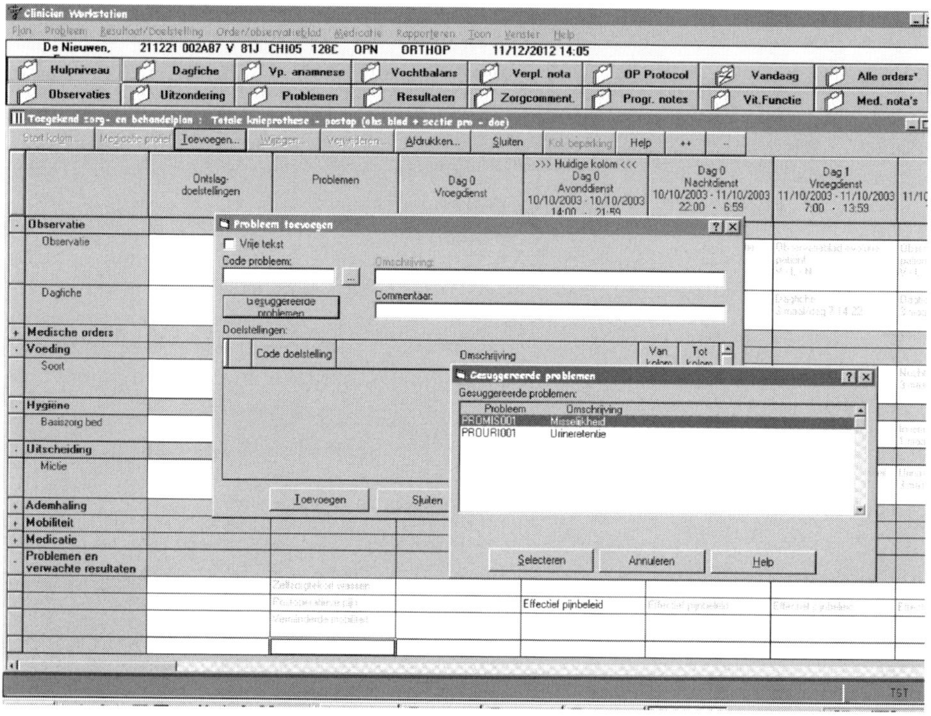

Care plan example

From the start of the project it was clear that such an evolution to clinical pathways is only possible in a WLAN environment with bedside access to the EPR [12]. The initial pilot on the department of traumatology was set-up with a number of distinctive goals in mind:

- Validate whether the software modules needed for care plan, observations, care plan merging, progress and outcome management were 'Nurseproof'.
- Test user-friendliness, feasibility and detect possible improvements.
- Evaluate the training schedules and workbooks in preparation of the bigger rollout.
- Validate the WLAN functionalities and set-up.

The department of traumatology was chosen as pilot environment, because the clinical pathways involved are rather straightforward. Also the effects of implementing them are well documented [13, 14]. For the pilot, 4 frequently used clinical pathways and a blank protocol were activated (hip prosthesis, knee prosthesis, trauma lower extremities, shoulder prosthesis). In total, about 20 clinical pathways have been parametrized in the system for traumatology (including the 5 used for the pilot).

Eight to twelve hours of training was given to each user, and temporary extra staffing and user support at the bedside were provided. During the first months of the pilot a lot of new functions were gradually phased in: nursing oriented anamnesis, preoperative checklist, nursing observations, care plan and charting.

2.2. Results

Plans are assigned to the patients according to the assessment of the physician in charge. As each plan is only an approximation of the care needed for that patient, the plans are individualised at the bedside. In case of mixed pathology or complex examinations, different care plans can easily be merged together. The system allows for care plans designed for dif-

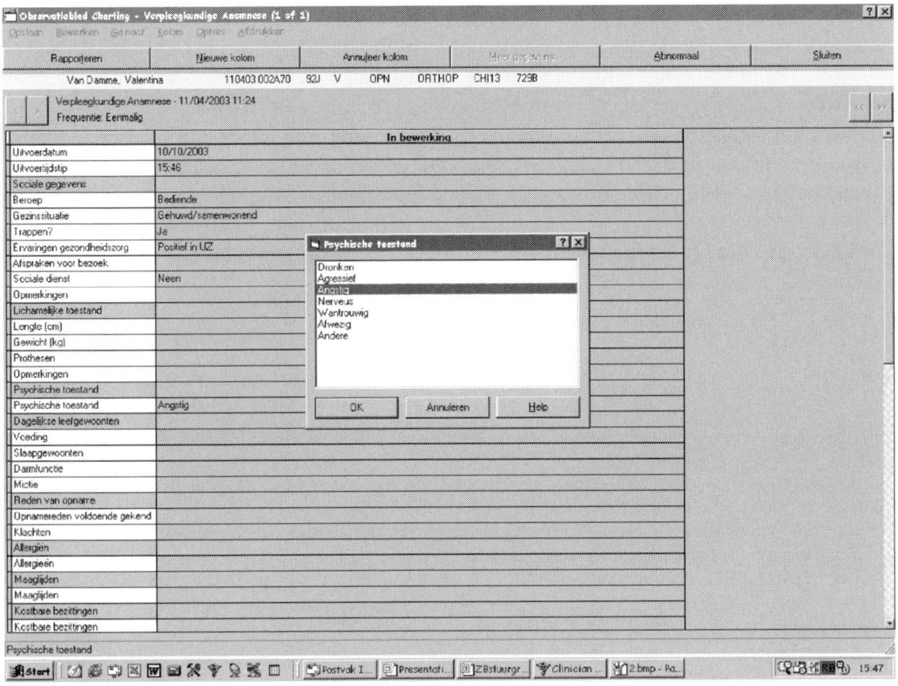

Observations

ferent departments to be merged together, e.g. after a patient transfer. Duplicates are automatically filtered out and/or presented to the user, e.g. in case different frequencies for one and the same service have to be merged.

Using questionnaires with open and closed questions and different evaluation rounds involving all users, the initial results showed a very good appreciation for the training, support and general acceptance of the new functionalities such as observations. Acceptance of the key care plan module was good although smaller software issues and sometimes shaky WLAN connection somewhat hampered the perceived user friendliness. Software issues included some printing problems, use of free text fields, changing of charting timestamps, order deletion, perceived complexity of some of the care plans etc.

The importance of detailed preparation, active involvement of the end users, a helpdesk which was able to give direct feedback and extensive support at the bedside are not to be underestimated here, lessons that were learnt the hard way during previous instalments of new EPR modules. Software related remarks were either solved by parametrization or taken up with Siemens, the EPR vendor, in order to further increase the user-friendliness or to patch up discovered glitches.

Obvious advantages of the care plan introduction include visualisation of the total care process, availability of all data within the EPR and better multidisciplinary coordination which all result in better patient care. In addition to this, continuous objective workload measurement becomes a reality.

3. Conclusions

In hospitals, the growing importance and maturity of electronic patient record systems and the gradual shift towards clinical pathways and integrated care, has necessitated access to the EPR from the bedside, only feasible in a wireless environment.

Although WLAN technology is still evolving much, the current status no longer prohibits a secure, hospital wide WLAN instalment, with a preference for 802.11b/g. However a number of smaller growing pains need to be addressed by implementers and by harmonisation of manufacturers' products. Possibilities for securing a WLAN have also reached an adequate level to minimize risk for sensitive medical data. Implementation still requires extensive domain knowledge for a correct and scalable set-up in the hospital environment.

The successful pilot implementation in the department of traumatology and the prepared roll-out to 5 more wards by the end of 2005 show that bedside integrated care plans have moved from the drawing board to reality thanks to the progression made in both EPR completeness and WLAN technology.

References

[1] Hilderink HG, ICT in nursing in Dutch hospitals, Studies in health technology and informatics, 2002; 93, pp. 83-8.
[2] Moloney R, A systematic review of the relationships between written manual nursing care planning, record keeping and patient outcomes, Journal of advanced nursing , 1999 Jul; 30 (1), pp. 51-7.
[3] Sengstack PP, CPOE systems: success factors and implementation issues, Journal of healthcare information management, 2004 Winter; 18 (1), pp. 36-45.
[4] www.ieee.org.
[5] Nash HO Jr, Wireless world. What are the options for today's health care facilities?, Health Facilities Management, 2003 Aug; Vol. 16 (8), pp. 25-30.
[6] www.citrix.com.
[7] Sims B, Deploying secure, reliable wireless LANs in the healthcare environment., Health Management Technologies, 2003 Apr; Vol. 24 (4), pp. 24, 27-9.
[8] Retterer J, Practice brief. Securing wireless technology for healthcare., American Health Information Management Association, 2004 May; Vol. 75 (5), pp. 56A-56D.
[9] www.oreillynet.com/lpt/a/408i.
[10] Berger R G, Computerized Physician Order Entry: Helpful or Harmful?, J Am Med Inform Assoc. 2004;11:100-103.
[11] King WJ, The effect of computerized physician order entry on medication errors and adverse drug events in pediatric inpatients., Pediatrics, 2003 Sep; Vol. 112 (3 Pt 1), pp. 506-9.
[12] Reynolds P, A Better Bedside Manner, Health Management Technology, 1074-4770, July 1, 2004, Vol. 25, Issue 7.
[13] Koval KJ , Clinical pathway for hip fractures in the elderly: the Hospital for Joint Diseases experience, Clin Orthop, 2004 Aug (425), pp. 72-81.
[14] Macario A, The effect of a perioperative clinical pathway for knee replacement surgery on hospital costs, Anesthesia and analgesia, 1998 May; 86 (5), pp. 978-84.

Contact address: tom.fiers@uzgent.be

A Nation-Wide Project for the Revision of the Belgian Nursing Minimum Dataset: From Concept to Implementation

Walter SERMEUS[a], *RN, PhD*, Koen VAN DEN HEEDE[a], *RN, MSc*,
Dominik MICHIELS[a], *RN, MSc*, Lucas DELESIE[a], *PhD*, Olivier THONON[b], *RN*,
Caroline VAN BOVEN[b], *RN*, Jean CODOGNOTTO[b], *RN* and Pierre GILLET[b], *MD, PhD*
[a]*Centre for Health Services Research, Catholic University of Leuven, Leuven, Belgium*
[b]*University Hospital of Liège, Liège, Belgium*

Abstract. This paper describes the process of revising the Belgian Nursing Minimum Data Set (NMDS). The study started in 2000. Implementation is planned from 2006. The project is divided in 4 major phases. The first phase (June – October 2002) implied the development of the conceptual framework based on literature review and secondary data-analysis. The Nursing Interventions Classification (NIC) was selected as framework for the revision of the NMDS. The second phase focused on the language development (November 2002 – September 2003) with panels of clinical experts (N=75) for six care programs. They indicated hospital financing, nurse staffing allocation and assessment of the appropriateness of hospitalization as priorities of a revised B-NMDS. A draft instrument with 84 variables, using NIC, was developed during this period. This leads to an alpha version of a revised NMDS. The third phase (October 2003 – December 2004) focused on the data collection and validation of the new tool. The new NMDS was tested on 158 nursing wards in 66 Belgian hospitals from December 2003 until March 2004. This test generated data for some 95.000 inpatient days. The interrater-reliability of the revised NMDS is tested. The criterion-related validity of the revised NMDS is compared with the actual NMDS. The discriminative power of the revised NMDS is tested to select the most relevant items for data collection. This will result in a beta version of revised NMDS in December 2004. The records of the revised NMDS are linked with the hospital discharge dataset and other mandatory datasets to integrate the revised NMDS in the broader health care management. The fourth phase (January – December 2005) will focus on information management.

Keywords. Nursing Minimum Data Set, Nursing care management, Nursing Interventions Classification, Diagnostic related groups

Introduction and Background

Belgium has a 15-year tradition of computer hospital data collection. It developed its Hospital Discharge Dataset (HDDS) in the 1980's and started full implementation in the 1990's. The dataset holds a set of relevant clinical information (primary and secondary diagnosis, procedures, length of stay, ..) for each patient discharged from an acute Belgian hospital. Also, Belgium is still one of the few countries that complement this HDDS with a nationwide uniform Nursing Minimum Dataset (NMDS) for a balanced sample of inpatient days. This NMDS data allows investigating nursing care and interventions and nurse staffing from 1987 onwards [1]. The mandatory registration resulted in an extensive dataset of more than 15 million selected in-patient days for some 6 million selected patients in all 2.500 nursing units in all Belgian hospitals. Nevertheless, the applications in clinical practice and health care management are still limited and touch only small part of the information available in the NMDS. The main application remains the use of the NMDS in determining some percentage points of the budget of the hospital. A few hospitals already use the data set to guide their staffing decisions. On the other hand, the evolutions in health care and nursing care in particular demand to update the NMDS. The Ministry of Public Health commissioned a research project to the Catholic university of Leuven and the University Hospital of Liège to revise the Belgian Nursing Minimum Dataset (NMDS) for six care programmes (cardiology, oncology, geriatrics, chronic care, paediatrics and intensive care) [2]. The study started in 2000 and envisage the implementation of the revised NMDS in 2006.

The revision aims to take into account the changes in nursing practice, the international development of nursing languages and classifications, the changes in healthcare management and the need for integration with the hospital discharge dataset.

Methodology and Procedure

To change is much more difficult than to start from scratch. For the revision of the B-NMDS a very strict plan is followed based on two main streams: 1) using panels of expert nurses and NMDS-coordinators to build the acceptability of the tool and 2) making use of existing and new empirical nursing data for developing a high-quality valid and reliable tool.

The project is divided in four major phases: 1) conceptualisation, 2) language development, 3) data collection and tool validation and 4) information management.
Each of these four consecutive phases will be discussed in this paper.

1. Phase I: Development of the Conceptual Framework

The first phase (June–October 2002) implied the development of the conceptual framework based on literature review and secondary data-analysis. The Nursing Interventions Classification (2nd Edition) or NIC was selected as framework for the revision of the NMDS. NIC is a comprehensive, research-based, standardised classification of interventions that nurses perform [3]. The 433 interventions in NIC (2nd Edition) are grouped into 27 classes and six domains for ease of use. This nursing language was selected for the revision of the Belgian NMDS because of strong validation work, the existence of the instrument in French and Dutch, the international use of the classification which allows further benchmarking and the fact the classification has also been tested before in Belgian home care [4].

2. Phase II: Language Development

The second phase focused on prioritizing future application domains and language development (November 2002–September 2003) with panels of clinical experts (N=75) for six care programs. Previous NMDS experience highlights the need to balance the considerable costs of registration with real-life improvements in nursing care and/or nursing management. It is only genuine to propose the registration of new data when the data of the existing NMDS or other related data sets seem insufficient to update existing indicators or to develop new ones.

First, the working groups had to concentrate on the selection of meaningful nursing care and nursing management indicators rather than to focus on individual data elements. They indicated hospital financing, nurse staffing allocation and assessment of the appropriateness of hospitalization as priorities of a revised NMDS. Secondly, the clinical experts of the 6 care programs selected the most relevant NIC interventions. All were studying the NIC classification. They selected the NIC interventions that are present in their current practice and indicated the relevance of each intervention for inclusion in a future nursing *minimum* dataset with the previous nominated priorities. In total 256 interventions, out of 433 were selected in at least 1 or more care programs. In a second phase, the results were presented to the clinical experts of each care program. Completeness of the items was discussed and the level of detail of measurement of the items was determined by the experts. All existing B-NMDS items (3) were listed and mapped into one framework: the NIC framework with domains, classes and interventions. NMDS items were put in the appropriate NIC domains and classes. NIC interventions were used to produce NMDS-items and response categories based on information of the six care program expert panels. This set of NMDS-items was pre-tested by the researchers in more then 3 wards per care programme and more than 15 different hospitals. This leaded to an alpha version of a revised NMDS with 87 variables.

3. Phase III: Pilot-Test and Tool Validation

The third phase (October 2003 – December 2004) focused on data collection, validation of the new tool and the integration with the HDDS.

3.1. Data Collection

Hospitals were solicited to participate in the study. This call for participation resulted in a total of 85 applying hospitals (69% of all Belgian acute hospitals) with 244 nursing wards. For feasibility reasons a selection was made based on well-defined selection criteria: equal regional and national distribution, balance between small and large hospitals, even number of private and public hospitals, teaching and non-teaching hospitals and an equal portion of wards for each care program. Hence, 66 Belgian hospitals with 158 nursing wards were selected to participate in this test. Each hospital nominated a project coordinator who is responsible for organization of education, data collection, data input and data transmission to the research teams. These coordinators had previous experience with the NMDS and with data handling.

The revised NMDS (alpha version) still uses a balanced sample of inpatient days and one-day hospitalisations. The alpha version of the revised NMDS was collected for about 95.000 inpatient days during thirty days and three registration periods (1-15 December 2003, 1-5 February 2004, 1-10 March 2004). The current NMDS- and HDDS-data for the patients included in this sample were also forwarded to the research team.

3.2. Reliability and Validity

Validity and reliability are important issues to consider when developing a new tool. In this study interrater reliability, criterion related-, construct-, face- and content validity are investigated. [5]

The *interrater-reliability* of the revised NMDS was tested on three points in time. Before each registration period the 66 coordinators were asked to score two written cases, describing the patient condition and nursing care given during one patient day. The six cases covered the six care programmes and included 60 of the 87 variables of the alpha version NMDS. The research team developed a gold-standard score per case. The scores of the coordinators were compared with the gold-standard scores.

The *criterion-related validity* of the revised NMDS is compared with the actual NMDS. This criterion-related validation approach, aims to objectively validate the revised NMDS in comparison with the actual NMDS. The rationale for this approach is that the similar elements of the revised tool should give at least the same level and detail of information as the previously validated actual NMDS. Firstly, the data collected with the revised tool during two of the three pilot-periods were coupled with the data of the available data from the actual NMDS. After a coupling based on common identifiers (patient number, date …), a database of 20.000 records was available for the comparison. After that, these coupled-data were recoded by the research team for every items of the 23 items of the actual NMDS, so that the data definitions in both datasets were as similar as possible. RIDIT-analysis [6] was used to standardize these variables and to aggregate them per nursing unit. The use of RIDITS makes it possible to assess the impact of the revised NMDS on the nursing profile of the nursing ward, the financial impact according to actual financing rules etc…. Finally, correlation of Spearman-rho and Kendall's tau b correlation coefficients were used to determine criterion-validity of the next B-NMDS. The analysis was performed on three levels: items, hospitals and care programs.

The discriminative power of the revised NMDS is tested to investigate the *construct-validity* of the tool. It is investigated how the items of the NMDS (alpha version) measure the expected constructs stated by the clinical experts during phase II of the project. This analysis-round aims to reduce the variables to a manageable number and withhold only those for nationwide registration, which are prerequisite to profiling nursing care for different pathology groups, nursing wards and hospitals. The registration of the revised NMDS follows the NIC$^{\text{2nd edition}}$-classes. Each NIC-class entails one or more variables. The data are analysed, with principal component analyses (CATPCA$^{©}$), in two steps using NIC as a framework. First, data are analysed per NIC-class. These *intra-class* analyses lead to the finding that variables are measuring the same latent variable, the aggregation of some (hierarchical) variables and the selection of variables with the highest discriminative power. In a second step, we repeated these analyses, using *inter-class* analyses to investigate the association of variables between classes. Both types of analysis were done per care program as well as on the total sample. This two-stepped analysis-round, will result in empirical based recommendations: registration guidelines, distinction between general, care-program specific and not-relevant variables.

The results from the interrater reliability, criterion related validity and construct-validity tests will be presented to the clinical experts (October – November 2004) to assure *face-validity* of the revised NMDS. They will discuss all the proposals of the researchers and suggest improvements based upon their clinical expertise and nursing care management experience. Based on these empirical test-results and the opinions of the clinical experts adjustments to the NMDS (alpha version) will be suggested.

A last component includes the cross-check of the selected NMDS variables with existing instruments in the literature to guarantee *content-validity*. Some specific updated NMDS variables should allow a patient classification system. This system will guide the allocation of staff within the different hospital wards on a daily and long-term basis. To assess the appropriateness of hospitalization we include the variables of the Belgian Appropriateness Evaluation Protocol in the updated B-NMDS. The NMDS-concepts will also be mapped with the NIC taxonomy and language. This will result in a beta version of revised NMDS in December 2004.

3.3. Integration of the NMDS with the HDDS

The NMDS-records are linked with the hospital discharge dataset. By linking both datasets we aim to develop a methodology to link the nursing data with diagnostic related groups (DRGs) in a logical and meaningful way and we also aim to measure the variability of nursing care per DRG. This data linking allows not only investigating the calender time which is important from an organisational perspective (e.g. nurse staffing, weekend-staffing...), but also the clinical time (e.g. pre-operative or post-op inpatient days for surgery patients; 5th , 10th chemotherapy inpatient days for oncology patients; etc.). As a result, the NMDS allows a managerial as well as a clinical perspective. A main application is a relative measurement of the type and intensity of nursing care per APR-DRG for each hospital and its care programmes. This will be done by linking the length of stay, the day of major surgical procedure, the day of chemotherapy,... from the HDDS with the nursing care and intervention data, staff and qualification data,... per day-of-stay from the new NMDS. The national data constitute the benchmark to delineate the frame of reference for each APR-DRG and to compare each hospital's specific situation. The methodology will be tested on a set of high-volume APR-DRGs. Identifying the key medical events and mapping the nursing data in this clinical timeframe, are key for evaluating each hospital's care processes. The analysis holds the evaluation of the consistency/variability of the nursing activity per day of stay, the degree of redundancy/uncertainty embedded in the HDDS and new NMDS datasets and the degree to which that both datasets allow meaningful monitoring of the whole care process. The study will help to understand how medical and nursing data interrelate. This understanding will be integrated in the final revised NMDS. The integration of medical and nursing data will lead to new applications for healthcare policy and management.

4. Phase IV: Developing Information Management Applications

The fourth phase (January – December 2005) focus on information management. The beta version of the Revised B-NMDS will be piloted in a small number of hospitals in a variety of departments and nursing wards to evaluate the external validity of the revised dataset. Linking the B-NMDS with the hospital discharge dataset will provide nursing profiles per DRG. Applications for hospital financing and nurse staff allocation will be developed. The B-NMDS will be incorporated in the evaluation of the appropriateness of stay in the hospital. Feedback and audit modules will be built. ICT-support in collecting and analysing the data will be developed. Adaptation in legislation to allow this revised data-collection will be prepared, to be ready for nation-wide implementation of the dataset in January 2006. The feasibility of running the fourth phase within the actual timeframe is now discussed with the Belgian Government.

Acknowledgments

The 'Actualization of the BNMDS' is supported and financed by the Belgian Federal Ministry of Social Affairs, Public Health and the Environment.

References

[1] Sermeus W., Delesie L., Van Landuyt J., Wuyts Y., Vandenboer G., Manna M. The Nursing Minimum Data Set in Belgium: a basic tool for the tomorrow's health care management. Leuven: Katholieke Universiteit Leuven; 1994.

[2] Sermeus W., Delesie L., Van den Heede K. Updating the Belgian Nursing Minimum Data Set: Framework and Methodology. In Roger France, F.H., Hasman, A. De Clerq, E. & De Moor, G. E-Health in Belgium and in the Netherlands: Proceedings of MIC 2002 (89-93). Amsterdam: IOS Press, 2002.

[3] McCloskey J.C., Bulechek G.M., Craft-Rosenberg M.C., Daley J., Denehey J., Glick O. et al. Nursing Interventions Classification (NIC) - second edition. St. Louis: Mosby-Year Book, Inc., 1996.

[4] De Vliegher K., Legiest E., Paquay L., Wouters L., Debaillie R., Geys L. Kerninterventies in de thuisverpleging. Wit-Gele Kruis, 2003.
[5] Polit D.F., Hungler B.P., Nursing research, Principles and methods – 5th edition, Lippincott Company.
[6] Sermeus W., Delesie L., Ridit analysis on ordinal data, Western Journal of Nursing Research, June 1996, v18 n3 p351 (9).

Address for correspondence

Prof. Walter Sermeus
Centre for Health Services Research
Catholic University of Leuven
Kapucijnenvoer 35/4
B-3000 Leuven
Belgium
Phone: +32 16336971
Fax: +32 16336970
e-mail: Walter.Sermeus@med.kuleuven.ac.be

From Patient Data to Information Needs

Loes BRAUN[a], Floris WIESMAN[b], Jaap VAN DEN HERIK[a], Arie HASMAN[b] and Erik KORSTEN[c]
[a]*Institute for Knowledge and Agent Technology, Universiteit Maastricht, P.O. Box 616, 6200 MD Maastricht, The Netherlands*
[b]*Department of Medical Informatics, Academic Medical Center, P.O. Box 22700, 1100 DE Amsterdam, The Netherlands*
[c]*Department of Anaesthesiology, Catharina-ziekenhuis, P.O. Box 1350, 5602 ZA Eindhoven, The Netherlands*

Abstract. The goal of this paper is to contribute to the improvement of the quality of care. For physicians, it is a problem that they are often not aware of gaps in their knowledge and the corresponding information needs. Our research aim is to resolve this problem by formulating information needs automatically. Based on these information needs, patient-specific literature can be retrieved. As a first step, we investigate how to model a physician's information needs. Thereafter, we design and analyse an approach to instantiate the model with patient data, resulting in information-need templates that are able to represent patient-specific information needs. Our experiments show that a physician's information needs can be modelled adequately and can be substantiated into patient-specific information needs. Since the number of formulated information needs is rather high, future research will focus on methods that restrict the set of automatically formulated information needs to a more specialized set.

Keywords. Medical Records Systems, Computerized, Information Storage and Retrieval, Quality of Health Care

Introduction

In our research[1], we investigate how to support physicians in the information-retrieval (IR) process, so as to improve the quality of care. We start with an example that precisely illustrates the need for patient-specific literature.

An 84-year-old woman was brought into the emergency department of a hospital, suffering from dyspnea and loss of consciousness. Five days earlier she had visited her general practitioner who diagnosed her with suspected respiratory tract infection and prescribed a drug called Clarithromycin. However, instead of improving, her condition worsened. In the hospital the diagnosis pneumonia was considered and she was treated accordingly, but without any effect. Upon her family's request, the patient was not admitted to the intensive care unit and she died one day after she was admitted to the hospital. Surprisingly, an autopsy revealed that the cause of death was not pneumonia, but a case of severe acute pancreatitis. The autopsy also revealed that the most plausible cause for the pancreatitis was the use of Clarithromycin, since pancreatitis is a (rare) side effect of the use of Clarithromycin [1].

Since the incidence of Clarithromycin-induced pancreatitis is quite low, it is understandable (but still undesirable) that the physician in the example above was not aware of this possible side effect. If the physician had performed a literature search in Medline on the side effects of Clarithromycin, he[2] probably would have found an article by Leibovitch, Levy, and Shoenfeld [2], in which another case of Clarithromycin-induced pancreatitis is discussed. If he had read this article, he probably would have ordered additional diagnostic tests to exclude pancreatitis (e.g., blood amylase) and he could have started the appropriate treatment immediately.

The reason why the physician did not perform a literature search is twofold. First, the physician was not aware of the fact that he needed information on the side effects of Clarithromycin. So, he had no incentive to search for information on the topic. Hence, we conclude that in this case there was an *implicit* information need. Second, even if the physician had been aware of his information need, he probably would not have had the time to perform a proper search action. The rapid growth of medical information sources and the complexity of the information spaces would impose too large a burden on a physician to retrieve information relevant to the specific patient.

The example above clearly illustrates that the retrieval of relevant, patient-specific literature is vital to the quality of care (cf. [3]). Various articles discuss IR systems that provide such literature (e.g., [4, 5, 6]); our research concurs with these articles. However, in our opinion the overall shortcoming of the systems mentioned in the articles above is that the degree of necessary interaction with the systems is too high. This is especially true in the area of making information needs explicit. Therefore, our main research objectives are (1) to investigate to what extent a physician's implicit information needs can be made explicit automatically, and (2) to implement our approach into a computer system supporting physicians in their daily work.

The article describes our approach in making a physician's implicit information needs explicit automatically. In Section 2 we describe how we determine a physician's information needs and how we model these needs. Section 3 presents our approach to formulate information needs regarding a specific patient, based on the patient data in the electronic patient record (EPR). In Section 4 experiments and results are discussed. Section 5 provides our conclusions and directions for future research.

1. Modelling a Physician's Information Needs

Our approach to make a physician's information needs explicit is to anticipate them. As a starting point for this process, we need a set of a physician's potential information needs. However, such a set can never be complete, since it is impossible to capture all of a physician's information needs. Moreover, a physician generates new information needs over time, which should be added to the set. This is hard to facilitate.

One solution is to build a *model* of a physician's information needs. As long as the model represents information needs on a more abstract level it can be considered complete, meanwhile anticipating future information needs. Modelling a physician's information needs involves two steps described below: (1) identifying a physician's information needs (Subsection 2.1) and (2) abstracting the identified information needs (Subsection 2.2).

1.1. Identifying a Physician's Information Needs

To identify a physician's information needs, we used two methods, viz. (1) a literature survey and (2) interviews. Both identification methods are briefly described below. Table 1 summarizes the sources, the identification domains, and the number of information needs identified.

Table 1. Number of information needs identified by a literature survey and interviews.

Identification method	Source	Identification domain	# INs identified
Literature survey	[7]	Outpatient care, inpatient care, internal medicine	16
	[8]	General practice, cardiology, pulmonology, allergology	77
	[9]	Family care	10
	[10]	Primary care	16
	[11]	Various	32
	[12]	Various	10
	[13]	Surgical care	2
	[14]	Primary care	8
Interviews		Anesthesiology	2
		Cardiology	1
		Neurology	0
		Pulmonology	3
		Surgery	3

In our literature survey, we searched for articles presenting information needs that are general, i.e., not specific for a particular group of physicians or for a particular geographical area. We found only eight such articles. This set of articles covered a large number of medical domains from which the information needs were identified. In total we arrived at 171 information needs.

To obtain a set of information needs that is as diverse as possible, we succeeded in interviewing five physicians in five different medical specialisms: (1) anaesthesiology, (2) cardiology, (3) neurology, (4) pulmonology, and (5) surgery. The physicians were interrogated by means of an interview scheme composed in advance. This led to 9 information needs.[3]

1.2. Abstracting the Identified Information Needs

The identified information needs are highly context-dependent, which may render them useless in another (different) context. To reduce context-dependency, we abstracted the information needs, so as to make them context-independent. For the abstraction we used an approach similar to the one used by Ely, Osheroff, and Ebell [9]. Hence, we replaced each medical concept in the information needs by its semantic type, which is a high-level description of the medical concept (e.g., the concept 'Pneumonia' has the semantic type DISEASE OR SYNDROME). We obtained the semantic types of the concepts from the Semantic Network of the Unified Medical Language System (UMLS) that comprises 135 types [15].

The abstraction resulted in a general class of information needs, called *information-need templates*. Some information needs resulted in the same information-need template. For example, *Does Norpace cause fatigue?* and *Does Clarithromycin cause high blood pressure?* both resulted in the information-need template *Does [CHEMICAL] cause [SIGN OR SYMPTOM]?* To obtain a proper *set* of information-need templates, we removed all doubles. Currently, the set comprises 167 information-need templates.

2. Converting Information-Need Templates into Information Needs

To formulate a patient-specific information need, an information-need template has to be instantiated with the patient's medical data. The data are acquired from the EPR of the specific patient. In our research we used the *Intensive Care Information System*,[4] used at the Intensive Care Unit of the Catharina-ziekenhuis in Eindhoven.

Our approach of converting an information-need template into a patient-specific information need comprises three steps described below.

(1) select EPR-queries that indicate the appropriate patient data[5] in the EPR,
(2) execute the selected EPR-queries: the desired data are extracted from the EPR, and
(3) instantiate the information-need template with the results of the executed queries.

In the first step, selecting the appropriate EPR-queries, we start determining which semantic types occur in the information-need template. To convert the information-need template into an information need, each of these semantic types has to be instantiated with patient data. Consequently, an EPR-query has to be selected for each semantic type in the information-need template. The EPR-queries are selected from a list of EPR-queries, formulated in advance. Each EPR-query in this list specifies how to find the patient data associated with the corresponding semantic type. Some high-level semantic types have subtypes, which should also be instantiated. We use the hierarchy within the UMLS Semantic Network to determine the subtypes of the high-level semantic types. For them queries are selected as well. Assume we have the following template:

What are the side effects of [CHEMICAL]?

Based on (1) the semantic type CHEMICAL, (2) the information structure of our EPR, and (3) the patient number of the specific patient, the EPR-query below is selected (the names of the database tables are in Dutch). Since the semantic type CHEMICAL has many subtypes (e.g., ORGANIC CHEMICAL and PHARMACOLOGIC SUBSTANCE), more EPR-queries are selected (viz. one query for each subtype), but for brevity, they are not presented here.

SELECT Medicijn FROM Medicatie WHERE PatientNummer=1234567890

In this approach, a difficulty occurs. Since EPR-systems are not yet standardized, EPRs from different EPR-systems have different information structures. Therefore, to adapt the system to another EPR-system, new EPR-queries have to be formulated. To facilitate easy adaptation, all potential EPR-queries for a specific EPR-system are specified in a model, which is runtime consulted by the system and can be easily reformulated.

The second step is to execute the selected queries to extract the desired patient data from the EPR. The actual query-execution process is handled by the database itself. Each result that an EPR-query returns for a semantic type is called an *instance* of that specific semantic type. Assume that our patient is taking three different medications (see Figure 1). Then, our EPR-query has three results and consequently, the semantic type CHEMICAL has three instances.

- *Clarithromycine*
- *Amoxi/Clavulaan*
- *Furosemide-iv*

There are two additional difficulties. First, the terms resulting from the EPR-query are in Dutch, whereas the information needs to be formulated have to be in English, because our system searches English literature databases. The translation of the terms is achieved by means of the UMLS Metathesaurus [15]. Second, some terms are not present in the UMLS Metathesaurus, because our EPR does not solely use standardized terms. Therefore, the UMLS SPECIALIST Lexicon [15] will be used to standardize these terms first.

The final step is to instantiate the information-need template with the data obtained from the EPR (the instances of the semantic types). We call an information-need template *applicable* (i.e., it can be instantiated with patient data) if each semantic type within the in-

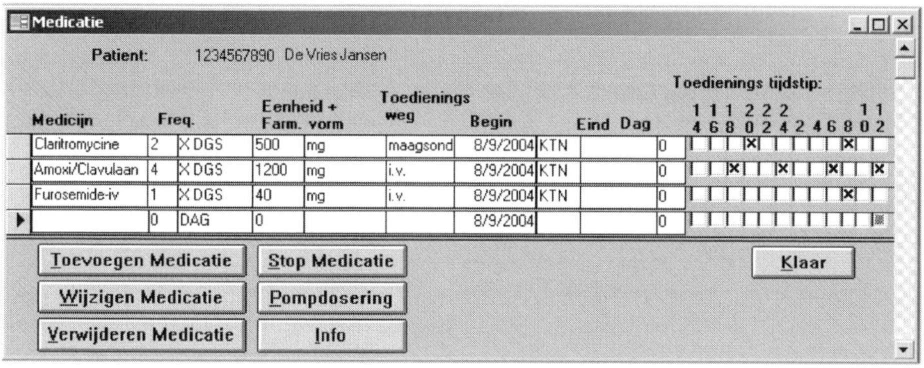

Figure 1. Interface of the Intensive Care Communication Information System, showing a patient's medication.

formation-need template has one or more instances. The template is instantiated by systematically replacing each semantic type by one of its instances, until all possible combinations are used. The total number of resulting information needs is the product of the numbers of instances of all semantic types in the template. For three instances (which are currently in Dutch) of the semantic type CHEMICAL, our information-need template is instantiated three times.

- *What are the side effects of Clarithromycine?*
- *What are the side effects of Amoxi/Clavulaan?*
- *What are the side effects of Furosemide-iv?*

If a literature search were conducted, based on the above information needs, patient-specific literature would be found. If not all semantic types have instances, the information-need template is not applicable and consequently it is not instantiated.

3. Experiments and Results

To establish the feasibility of our approach for instantiating information-need templates, we let our system formulate information needs based on the EPRs of 90 patients. Each EPR contained information about *all* hospital admissions (in the hospital under consideration) of a specific patient. We used our complete set of 167 information-need templates. For each patient, our experiment resulted in a set of information needs. We divided the number of formulated information needs into four categories, viz. (i) no information needs, (ii) a manageable number of information needs, (iii) a hardly manageable number of information needs, and (iv) and unmanageable number of information needs. We placed each patient in one of these categories, based on the number of formulated information needs associated with the patient (see Figure 2).

As can be seen in Figure 2, the total number of information needs is quite high for most patients. If a literature search were conducted for all these information needs, the set of retrieved literature would be unmanageably high. Since we do not want to overload physicians with literature, the number of information needs for which literature is retrieved should be restricted. In the ideal situation, all patients would be in category 1-100 information needs.

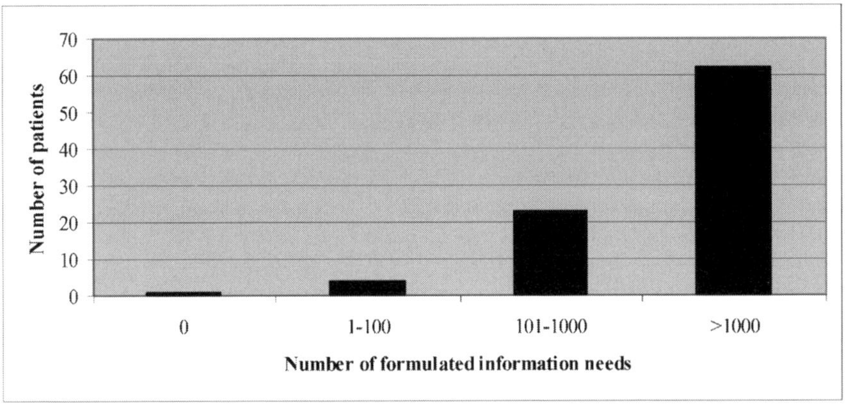

Figure 2. Number of patients for which a specific number of information needs is formulated.

4. Conclusions and Future Research

The investigations with physicians, described in Subsection 2.1, showed that we succeeded in identifying a physician's potential information needs and in modelling them into 167 information-need templates by using 135 semantic types (Subsection 2.2).

In Section 3 we designed an approach to convert information-need templates into patient-specific information needs by taking patient data into account. When these information needs are used as a starting point for a literature search, a physician can be provided with relevant and patient-specific medical literature. From the experiments, we may conclude that our approach is adequate and can be generalized to other EPR-systems, as long as they use a clear information structure. In Section 3 we mentioned that Dutch non-standardized terms in the EPR present a problem to our approach. A part of our future research will concentrate on solving this problem.

The number of automatically formulated information needs per patient is still high (Section 4). Since a high number of information needs will lead to a large amount of retrieved literature, physicians would be overloaded with information. So, our approach is not yet sufficiently adequate. To improve the approach, the number of information needs for which literature is retrieved should be restricted. Another part of our future research will focus on this restriction by taking two additional parameters into account. The first parameter is the *usefulness of the patient data*. In our experiment, data from all hospital admissions (in the hospital under consideration) were used to generate information needs, whereas only patient data that are relevant to the patient's current problem are important. Therefore, it is essential to distinguish between useful and non-useful data. In general, the current admission will provide the most useful data. However, not all data from the current admission might be useful. For example, when a physician has already selected chemotherapy as the appropriate treatment for a lung-cancer patient, he may be assumed not to have information needs concerning the selection of a treatment, e.g., *What is the treatment for lung cancer for this patient?* Yet, he might still have information needs concerning the execution of the selected treatment, e.g., *How high is the dose of chemotherapy for lung cancer for this patient?* The second parameter is the *specialism of the physician*. Since a physician's information needs are probably connected to his specialism, we might ignore several information needs, because they are not linked to the physician's specialism. Ignoring the information needs is solely based on the patient data with which the corresponding information-need templates were instantiated. As information-need templates contain no patient data, templates cannot be ignored in advance. A series of experiments may clarify whether the two parameters are appropriate filters for the number of information needs.

Endnotes

[1] This research is part of the MIA project (Medical Information Agent), which is funded by NWO (grant number 634.000.021).
[2] For brevity we will use the pronoun 'he' ('his') where 'he or she' ('his or her') is meant.
[3] Since we have to search English literature and several information needs were in Dutch, we translated the Dutch information needs into English.
[4] Intensive Care Informatie Systeem, Version 2.8. INAD Computers & Software B.V. Eindhoven, Werkgroep ICIS Afd. Intensive Care, Dienst Informatie Voorziening, Catharina-ziekenhuis Eindhoven.
[5] All patient data used in the examples of Section 3 are fictitious.

References

[1] B.J.J.W. Schouwenberg and J. Deinum. Acute pancreatitis after a course of clarithromycin. *The Netherlands Journal of Medicine*, 61(7):266–267, 2003.
[2] L. Leibovitch, Y. Levy, and Y. Shoenfeld. Pancreatitis induced by Clarithromycin. *Annals of Internal Medicine*, 125(8):701, October 1996.
[3] S. Gamble. Hospital libraries enhance patient care and save money. *Journal of the Alberta Association of Library Technicians*, 23(2):10–12, 1996.
[4] R.A. Miller, L. Jamnback, N.B. Giuse, and F.E. Masarie. Extending the capabilities of diagnostic decision support programs through links to bibliographic searching: Addition of 'canned MeSH logic' to the Quick Medical Reference (QMR) program for use with Grateful Med. In P. Clayton, editor, *Proceedings of the Fifteenth Annual Symposium on Computer Applications in Medical Care (SCAMC), Washington, DC*, pages 150–155, New York, NY, 1991. McGraw-Hill, Inc.
[5] R. Rada, J. Barlow, D. Bijstra, J. Potharst, P. de Vries Robbé, and P. Zanstra. OAR: Open architecture for reasoning applied to connection patient records to medical literature. In J. Noothoven van Goor and J.P. Christensen, editors, *Advances in Medical Informatics*, pages 287–294, Amsterdam, The Netherlands, 1992. IOS Press.
[6] E.M. van Mulligen. UMLS-based access to CPR data. *International Journal of Medical Informatics*, 53(2–3):125–131, 1999.
[7] R.J. Cucina, M.K. Shah, D.C. Berrios, and L.M. Fagan. Empirical formulation of a generic query set for clinical information retrieval systems. In V. Patel, R. Rogers, and R. Haux, editors, *MedInfo2001. Proceedings of the 10th World Congress on Medical Informatics, London, United Kingdom*, pages 181–185, Amsterdam, The Netherlands, 2001. IOS Press.
[8] P.F. de Vries Robbé, W.P.A. Beckers, and P.E. Zanstra. *MEDES. Het prototype*. Onderzoeksgroep Medische Informatie- en Besliskunde, Academische Ziekenhuis Groningen, Groningen, The Netherlands, 1988. (In Dutch).
[9] J.W. Ely, J.A. Osheroff, and M.H. Ebell. Analysis of questions asked by family doctors regarding patient care. *British Medical Journal*, 319(7206):358–361, 1999.
[10] P.N. Gorman. Information needs of physicians. *Journal of the American Society for Information Science*, 46(10):729–736, 1995.
[11] H.G.L.M. Grundmeijer, K. Reenders, and G.E.H.M. Rutten, editors. *Het Geneeskundig Proces. Van Klacht naar Therapie*. Elsevier Gezondheidszorg, Maarssen, The Netherlands, 1999. (In Dutch).
[12] R.N. Jerome, N.B. Giuse, K.W. Gish, N.A. Sathe, and M.S. Dietrich. Information needs of clinical teams: analysis of questions received by the clinical informatics consult service. *Bulletin of the Medical Library Association*, 89(2):177–185, 2001.
[13] M.C. Reddy, W. Pratt, P. Dourish, and M.M. Shabot. Asking questions: Information needs in a surgical intensive care unit. In I.S. Kohane, editor, *Proceedings of the Annual AMIA Symposium (AMIA'02), San Antonio, Texas*, pages 647–651, 2002.
[14] R. Smith. What clinical information do doctors need? *British Medical Journal*, 313(7064):1062–1068, 1996.
[15] U.S. National Library of Medicine. Unified Medical Language System, 2003. http://www.nlm.nih.gov/research/umls/.

Address for correspondence:

Drs. L.M.M. Braun, Institute for Knowledge and Agent Technology, Universiteit Maastricht, P.O. Box 616, 6200 MD Maastricht, The Netherlands, L.Braun@cs.unimaas.nl

Quality of Care Assessment using GPs' Electronic Patient Records: Do We Need Data from Home Visits?

Hans VANDENBERGHE[a], Viviane VAN CASTEREN[a], Pascale JONCKHEER[b], Marie-France LAFONTAINE[a] and Etienne DE CLERCQ[c]
[a]*Scientific Institute of Public Health (IPH), unit of Epidemiology*
J. Wytsmanstraat 14, 1050 Brussels, Belgium
h.vandenberghe@iph.fgov.be
[b]*Société Scientifique de Médecine Générale (SSMG), Brussels, Belgium*
[c]*Health Systems Research (HSR), School of Public Health,*
Université Catholique de Louvain (UCL), Brussels, Belgium

Abstract. The paper tackles the topic of collecting data from home visits using the electronic patient record (EPR) of general practitioners (GPs), in a context with a high proportion of home visits in primary care. Since data from home visits, representing about 40% of GPs' consultations in Belgium, are rather scarcely recorded in the EPR, we wanted to study the impact of not taking into account home visits for quality assessment in primary care. Five quality indicators, which measured the accordance of the delivered care with guidelines on the management of osteoarthritis, were compared between a pooled database (consultations and home visits) and a restricted database (after removal of home visits). Our findings suggest that removing home visits from a database collected from primary care may provide a slight modification of the estimate of the quality of care, whereas conclusions on quality improvement remain relatively stable. Quality of care assessment with the EPR of GPs seems not to be dramatically hampered by the poor recording rate of home visits in the EPR.

Keywords. Primary Health Care, Computerized Patient Records, Data Collection Method, Home Visits, Quality of Care Assessment

Introduction

There is an emerging trend to conduct studies of quality assessment in health care using data obtained from electronic patient records (EPRs), both in hospital [1] and in primary care [2-5]. Obtaining information from EPRs for research on quality of care has encountered, however, some obstacles, such as the problem of missing data in the EPR [6]. Parameters need to be entered first by general practitioners (GPs) into the EPR before they can be extracted from that EPR. But GPs record data in the EPR when they think they are useful for daily health care practice and research objectives are not on their mind. Hence, the situation where parameters needed for quality assessment are missing in the electronic patient record is frequently occurring. It is, for instance, known that data from home visits are recorded much less in the EPR than are consultation data [7]. Devices are being developed in order to bridge that gap (e.g. PDA, tablet PC) but are still unsatisfactory in their use. In a context with various EPR software systems on the market such as in Belgium (currently about twenty different systems) bridging that gap is even more difficult. We have also to keep in mind that in Belgium many GPs' contacts are home visits (47% in 1999; slightly decreasing over the last years) [8].

The challenge for health services researchers is now to evaluate the usefulness of data obtained from the EPR for research, by taking account of these obstacles. Given the poor recording rate for data from home visits in the EPR, one of the questions posed is whether we need data from home visits for quality of care assessment, anyway. Currently, we have no knowledge of a study having explored that aspect.

In this paper the research question is whether the information on the quality of care for osteoarthritis in general practice is significantly different when home visits are not taken into account compared to when they are. We believe this question is of high importance for the implementation of data collection networks with the EPR for quality of care assessment in general practice in countries where GPs' involvement in home visiting is substantial. In one study Belgium was identified as on the top of 18 European countries for GPs' involvement in home visiting, but also other countries had a relative high number of visits per week [9].

If the answer to the above question is negative, then, in a first stage, the obstacle of the poor recording rate of home visits in the EPR can be overcome very easily, by leaving out data from home visits from the analysis for quality assessment.

1. Methods

1.1. Data Collection

At the Scientific Institute of Public Health (IPH) and with the collaboration of the two scientific associations of GPs in Belgium and a university, a cross-sectional study on the medical management of osteoarthritis (OA) in general practice was conducted in 2001 and repeated in 2003, respectively called the first and the second phase. In both phases, data on prescribed drugs were collected from patients with osteoarthritis of 60 years or above, who contacted their GP over a period of five weeks, respectively from 05/02/2001 till 11/03/2001 in the first phase and from 10/03/2003 till 06/04/2003 in the second phase. Patients were included in the study independently of the place of contact, which was also registered during both phases (consultation at the surgery or home visit). GPs could choose for collecting data either on paper registration sheets or through an extraction of data from the electronic patient record, but the set of parameters collected was equal for both data collection methods. Details about the electronic data collection method have been described elsewhere [10].

1.2. Quality Indicators

In 2001 and 2003, we calculated five prescribing indicators, which were designed to measure the accordance of the delivered care with the recommendations of evidence-based guidelines for the treatment of osteoarthritis (quality indicators). Guidelines suggest that OA treatment should not start with drugs. When a drug therapy is decided, paracetamol – a simple painkiller without side effects at the recommended dose – is preferred to non-steroidal anti-inflammatory drugs (NSAID). Because the latter have negative side effects, especially on the gastro-intestinal and renal systems, repeat prescriptions should be avoided. Finally, the added value of the last generation of NSAIDs (COXIBS) is still under debate in the literature. The indicators assessed respectively, whether or not there was a

Table 1. Quality indicators.

Indicator	Numerator	Denominator
Drug prescription	Patients with a drug prescription for osteoarthritis in the past month	All patients with osteoarthritis
Paracetamol	Patients who were prescribed paracetamol	All patients with a drug prescription for osteoarthritis in the past month
NSAID	Patients who were prescribed an NSAID	All patients with a drug prescription for osteoarthritis in the past month
Coxib	Patients who were prescribed a coxib	All patients who received an NSAID for osteoarthritis in the past month
Repeated	Patients who received a repeat prescription	All patients who received an NSAID for osteoarthritis in the past month

drug prescription for OA during the past month, the type of drug and the type of NSAID prescribed for OA during the past month and whether or not the NSAID prescription was a repeat prescription (Table 1).

1.3. Analysis

In order to respond to the research question, we took three steps in the data analysis.

In *step one*, only data obtained from GPs collecting data through the EPR-method were taken and comparisons were made for the five quality indicators between the database containing data from consultations at the surgery and home visits (pooled database) and the database after removal of home visits (restricted database). The comparisons were made for both phases of the study, separately.

We then, as a *second step*, switched to the data obtained from GPs having collected data on paper sheets (the paper group) and carried out the same comparison for both phases.

In the *third step*, we made a longitudinal assessment of change in quality (difference in prescribing indicators between the first and the second phase of the study) and compared the results between the pooled and restricted database. We did this analysis only with data from the paper group. We made adjusted estimates of change for the five indicators using logistic regression with year of data collection, patient age, sex and severity of disease as independent factors.

Our hypothesis was that results probably would not differ a lot between the compared databases (before and after removal of home visits) for data obtained with the EPR-method since a minority of the contacts will be home visits (due to poor data recording), while this is very likely not the case for data obtained with paper registration sheets. By taking the data from the paper group, with an expected higher proportion of home visits, we simulate the ideal situation where EPRs contain a large amount of data from home visits. Therefore, we proceeded to the third step in the analysis only for the paper group (the ideal situation).

The analyses were restricted to data from GPs who participated in both phases and only the first contact with the patient was retained in the case a patient was seen several times in the registration period. We used SPSS 11.5 for all analyses.

2. Results

Hundred eighty-three (183) GPs contributed data from both phases to the study. Respectively in the first and the second phase data was collected for 7843 (5711 in the paper group, 2132 in the EPR-group) and 7456 (paper: 5272, EPR: 2184) patients with osteoarthritis. The proportion of home visits slightly decreased between the two periods (50% in 2001 versus 48% in 2003).

Table 2. Comparison of quality indicators, pooled database (consultations at the surgery and home visits) versus restricted database (home visits removed): EPR, 2001.

Indicator	Pooled database		Restricted database		P of Chi²
	N	%	N	%	
Drug prescription	673	31.6	443	28.6	0.052
Paracetamol	136	20.2	74	16.7	0.143
NSAID	424	63.0	300	67.7	0.106
Coxib	62	14.6	46	15.3	0.791
Repeated	226	53.3	158	52.7	0.866

Table 3. Comparison of quality indicators, pooled database (consultations at the surgery and home visits) versus restricted database (home visits removed): EPR, 2003.

Indicator	Pooled database		Restricted database		P of Chi²
	N	%	N	%	
Drug prescription	738	33.8	528	31.6	0.158
Paracetamol	148	20.1	92	17.4	0.239
NSAID	489	66.3	350	66.3	0.992
Coxib	122	24.9	96	27.4	0.419
Repeated	260	53.2	193	55.1	0.572

Table 4. Comparison of quality indicators, pooled database (consultations at the surgery and home visits) versus restricted database (home visits removed): PAPER, 2001.

Indicator	Pooled database		Restricted database		P of Chi²
	N	%	N	%	
Drug prescription	3541	62.0	1415	60.5	0.207
Paracetamol	1134	32.0	388	27.4	0.002*
NSAID	2131	60.2	944	66.7	0.003*
Coxib	421	19.8	200	21.2	0.362
Repeated	1055	49.5	450	47.7	0.347

Step one:

Respectively in the first and the second phase, only 27% and 24% of the contacts with patients in the EPR group were home visits. After removal of these home visits, the five compared indicators did not change with statistical significance, not in 2001 (Table 2), nor in 2003 (Table 3).

Step two:

In the paper group, 59% of the patients included in 2001 were seen during home visits. The proportion of patients taking paracetamol and those taking NSAID both changed significantly after removal of home visits from the database (Table 4). In 2003 the proportion of home visits was 58%. The results for drug prescription, paracetamol and NSAID were significantly different between the pooled and restricted database (Table 5).

Table 5. Comparison of quality indicators, pooled database (consultations at the surgery and home visits) versus restricted database (home visits removed): PAPER, 2003.

Indicator	Pooled database		Restricted database		P of Chi^2
	N	%	N	%	
Drug prescription	3692	70.1	1476	66.3	0.001*
Paracetamol	1771	47.9	630	42.7	0.001*
NSAID	2011	54.4	912	61.7	< 0.001*
Coxib	713	35.5	332	36.4	0.620
Repeated	1163	57.8	497	54.5	0.092

Table 6. Logistic regression for change in 2001–2003, pooled database versus restricted database: PAPER.

Indicator	Pooled database		Restricted database	
	Adjusted* OR change	95% CI	Adjusted OR change	95% CI
Drug prescription	1.49	(1.37 – 1.62)	1.31	(1.16 – 1.49)
Paracetamol	1.90	(1,72 – 2,10)	1.97	(1.68 - 2.31)
NSAID	0.82	(0.74 – 0.90)	0.80	(0.69 – 0.94)
Coxib	2.30	(1.99 – 2.66)	2.15	(1.74 – 2.65)
Repeated	1.43	(1.26 – 1.62)	1.35	(1.12 – 1.63)

* adjusted for patient age, sex and severity of osteoarthritis

Step three:

As already mentioned this step is only carried out in the paper group. When the results were compared between both databases, the adjusted odds ratios for change between both years were at the same side of the 1-value, although the values of the odds ratios changed slightly (Table 6). In the pooled database, the proportion of patients with a drug prescription for OA in the past month had increased between 2001 and 2003. There was also an increase for paracetamol use, coxib use and repeat prescriptions. On the contrary, the proportion of patients with an NSAID prescription had decreased. The same observations could be made in the restricted database.

3. Discussion

As expected, home visits were widely underestimated (27% in 2001 and 24% in 2003) in the EPR group. This may be due to poor recording of home visits data in the EPR. The high rate of home visits in the paper group (59% in 2001, 57.7% in 2003) compared to that of the literature [8] (47% in 1999) could be explained by the investigated population in this study (the elderly).

When home visits were removed from the pooled database obtained through EPR-extraction, the five indicators showed no statistically significant change in their results, in both phases of the study. This observation could lead us to conclude that quality assessment for osteoarthritis in general practice with EPR-data does not need to include data from home visits. However, our observation in the EPR-group may be due to both relatively small sample sizes (and hence a small power to be able to find differences) and the relatively small contribution of home visits to the pooled database.

Therefore, we carried out the same analysis with the database obtained by paper registration sheets (the paper group), in order to simulate the situation when home visits are well recorded in the EPR and when many data are obtained through the EPR. In this way, we rule out the two factors (small contribution of home visits and small sample size) that could confound our findings.

In the paper group, the observation is somewhat different. In both phases, two indicators (proportion of patients on paracetamol, proportion of patients on NSAID) did not have the same results when home visits were removed from the pooled database. Only in 2003, this was the case for the first indicator (drug prescriptions).

When only data are used from consultations at the surgery, the cross-sectional assessment of the quality of care for osteoarthritis provided a slightly underestimated judgement. Indeed, when home visits were removed, the proportion of paracetamol users (indicator of "good" quality) and NSAID users (indicator of "bad" quality), respectively, decreased and increased. A possible explanation could be that patients seen during home visits have a relatively higher probability of multi-morbidity and therefore a more conservative drug treatment is applied (drugs with less side effects). Further research is required to explain our findings.

The direction of the trends in prescription for osteoarthritis was equal after removal of the home visits (increase in drug prescriptions, paracetamol use, coxib use and repeat prescriptions and decrease of NSAID), although the extent of the trends was slightly different (we do not have a statistical measure of difference between the odds ratios). This means that the overall conclusions for quality improvement (trends for paracetamol and NSAID supported by the guidelines and trends against recommendations in guidelines for drug prescriptions, coxibs and repeat prescriptions) were the same independently of whether or not home visits were included.

Although this study is about a specific part of general practice (the management of osteoarthritis in the elderly) and in a context of high GP involvement in home visiting we believe it may be of interest to researchers using EPR-data from general practice in other countries with the same context regarding the importance of home visits in primary care and the same difficulties to catch data related to home visits. Even in Belgium, where more than 40% of GPs' contacts are home visits, these contacts may sometimes be withdrawn without dramatically hampering the results of quality of care assessment studies.

4. Conclusions

Quality of care assessment with data obtained from the EPR of GPs becomes more widespread. However, there are still many obstacles to be overcome, amongst them the cumbersome inclusion of data from home visits in these EPRs. In this paper the aim was to test the impact of leaving out home visits from the research database on the results of quality of care assessment studies.

Analyses of drug prescription data from a study on the management of osteoarthritis in the elderly have shown that a cross-sectional assessment of the quality of care may be slightly different when home visits are excluded (the data suggested, quite unexpectedly, an underestimation of quality when home visits were removed). On the contrary, the assessment of quality improvement (change in quality indicators over time) did not lead to different conclusions between whether or not home visits were included.

By using a large database with a high proportion of home visits, we have simulated the situation where EPRs contain a large amount of data from home visits and hence the above conclusions can be extrapolated towards the future. Including data from home visits in the EPR should not necessarily be considered as high priority for carrying out studies of quality improvement in general practice, using data obtained from EPRs.

References

[1] Bates DW, Pappius EM, Kuperman GJ, Sittig D, Burstin H, Fairchild D et al. Measuring and improving quality using information systems. Medinfo 1998; 9 Pt 2:814-818.
[2] Bierma-Zeinstra SM, Lipschart S, Njoo KH, Bernsen R, Verhaar J, Prins A et al. How do general practitioners manage hip problems in adults? Scand J Prim Health Care 2000; 18(3):159-164.
[3] Donoghue JM, Tylee A. The treatment of depression: prescribing patterns of antidepressants in primary care in the UK. Br J Psychiatry 1996; 168(2):164-168.
[4] Hooker RC, Cowap N, Newson R, Freeman GK. Better by half: hypertension in the elderly and the 'rule of halves': a primary care audit of the clinical computer record as a springboard to improving care. Fam Pract 1999; 16(2):123-128.
[5] Kirk SA, Campbell SM, Kennell-Webb S, Reeves D, Roland MO, Marshall MN. Assessing the quality of care of multiple conditions in general practice: practical and methodological problems. Qual Saf Health Care 2003; 12(6):421-427.
[6] Prins H, Kruisinga FH, Buller HA, Zwetsloot-Schonk JH. Availability and usability of data for medical practice assessment. Int J Qual Health Care 2002; 14(2):127-137.
[7] Hamilton WT, Round AP, Sharp D, Peters TJ. The quality of record keeping in primary care: a comparison of computerised, paper and hybrid systems. Br J Gen Pract 2003; 53(497):929-933.
[8] De Maeseneer J, De Prins L, Heyerick JP. Home visits in Belgium: a multivariate analysis. European Journal of General Practice 1999; 5(1):11-14.
[9] Boerma WGW, Groenewegen PP. GP home visiting in 18 european countries. Adding the role of health system features. Eur J Gen Pract 2001; 7:132-137.
[10] De Clercq E, Vandenberghe H, Jonckheer P, Bastiaens H, Lafontaine MF, Van Casteren V. Assessment of a three-year experience with a Belgian Primary Care data Network. Stud Health Technol Inform 2002; 93:163-169.

Exploitation of Electronic Medical Records Data in Primary Health Care. Resistances and Solutions. Study in Eight Walloon Health Care Centres

Marc VANMEERBEEK, *MD*
Département de Médecine générale, Université de Liège
Domaine du Sart Tilman (Bât. B23) - CHU - 4000 Liège, Belgium

Abstract. *Introduction*: The Electronic Medical Records (EMR), used every day for primary health care may constitute an instrument for gathering locally usable data to improve the quality of care and, on a larger scale, be a basis of epidemiological data. In spite of a policy of promotion of the EMR made by the Federation of French-speaking Belgian "Medical Houses", its use remains very marginal.

Methods: Eight Medical Houses, motivated by computerization of medical records have been met. Quantitative indicators of use of the EMR have been assessed. A qualitative assessment of the resistances to computerization, and solutions which can be brought, has been realized through the technique of the nominal group.

Results: The use of the EMR remains slight, allowing for exceptions. The proposed solutions could be put together in 5 categories : ethics, training, search for sense, practice and interdisciplinarity.

Discussion: The practitioners are willing to computerize if they get immediate advantages (knowledge of their patients and their team operating). They expressed the need of having a tool easy to use, that doesn't make them lose time and that has respect for their specificity of work and organization (interdisciplinary and self-managed teams). They expressed the need of an external support, under the form of adapted training and supervision for the data management. Ethical concerns (security, data transfer, place of the computer in the relationship with the patient) are surprisingly not present enough.

Keywords. MeSH: Belgium, Group Practice, Prepaid, Electronic Medical Records, Databases, Software design, Attitude to Computers, Qualitative research

Introduction

The use of structured records for each patient in primary health care makes it possible to follow his story for a length of time and, in theory, to work towards giving him the most appropriated care. The epidemiological database which can be gained from the aggregation of those individual records is considerable and can be valorised [1, 2], and constitutes the base of a Health Information System.

The Federation of French-speaking Belgian Medical Houses (FMH) has been developing for some years an interdisciplinary Electronic Medical Record (EMR). It is established in 40 French-speaking teams and 6 Dutch-speaking ones. The professional's motivation to enter in an approach of gathering clinical data from the consultations is determining for the durability of the action and the quality of the data. In spite of some different encouragements and personalized teams meetings [3], the use of EMR seems to remain very slight, and the quality of some collected data very insufficient in the sight of what could be done [4].

The objectives of this work were:

- To assess of indicators of the present use of the FMH's EMR.
- To define, with the participation of the users, the content of an action program for Medical Houses with having in mind the removing of the resistances to the data collection in Primary Care through the use of EMR.

1. Methods

1.1. Setting

A two hours meeting on their workplace has been proposed to eight Walloons teams who , at their demand, had enjoyed in 2002-2003 actions of promotion of the use of EMR. All accepted. Those teams had been on an inclusive basis financed by the insurance companies, and they worked in self-management. The used software (PRICARE 3.2.23) records the meetings with the patients under the form of contacts bound to one or more episodes of care (ICPC-1 classified).

The meetings (May 2004) consisted, on the one hand, in a quantitative measure on their database and, on the other hand, in a qualitative estimation of the resistances on the use of the EMR and the solutions which could be brought. The technique of the nominal group, validated for problem identification and needs, and for hierarchical organization of solutions has been used [5, 6]. In order to work on a positive formulation of the problems, the question was focused on the considered solutions: **"How can we beat the present blockings to valorise the data our EMR can contain ?"**

1.2. Quantitative Measures

Three quantitative indicators of the use of the EMR have been measured:

- The proportion of patient met in 2003 with at least 1 episode of care in their record, which expressed the minimum frequency of use of the EMR.
- The number of episodes per patient during 2003, per profession, expressing the intensity of use of the EMR.
- The comparison of the number of (sub)-contact noted in the EMR (recorded clinical activities) with the number of performed acts (real activity), per professional area.

Those indicators have been previously standardized in 4 reference teams (further called REF1 to REF4). The last two indicators have been confronted with the measures of Okkes et al. [7] for the doctors.

1.3. Qualitative Analysis

The content of discussions and votes in nominal group have been fully transcribed. The priority rank of the verbatims of each team has been calculated immediately by totalising the points and has been discussed with the participants. The semantic content has been analysed later, and closely related with the objective data of the databases.

2. Results

2.1. Indicators of Use of the EMR

2.1.1. Proportion of Patients met in 2003 with at least One Episode of Care in their Record

One team (Nr 7) has a very high frequency of use of the EMR (96%) and 2 others (Nr 4 and 6) have surpassed the stage of isolated testing and are probably rising users (61% and 49%). The others have an occasional use or isolated users in their team (0.1 to 12%).

2.1.2. Number of Episodes Created by Patient during 2003

The intensivity of use varies between 2.3 and 3.6 new episodes per patient and per year in the reference teams, a little more than in the measures by Okkes (1.3 to 2.5 new episode per year, according to different countries). The two rising teams are also in that standard and team 7 exceeds it (4 new episode per year).

2.1.3. Professions who Incode Episodes

Everywhere, the doctors are responsible for the creation of more than 95% of the episodes, except in one team where physiotherapists does it nearly exclusively.

2.1.4. Proportion of Sub-Contacts with Patients Noted in the EMR: Table 1

Only team Nr 7 uses EMR to note consultations in every professional area. The behaviour of practitioners of the reference teams is rather heterogeneous, specially by the paramedical personal. A part of the doctors record more than in the measures by Okkes et al.

2.2. Analysis of Content of the Nominal Groups

We met 57 practitioners, among them 24 doctors, 12 receptionists, 6 physiotherapists, 6 administrative clerks, 5 nurses, 2 psychologists and 2 social workers.

The 178 verbatims produced by the 8 groups after the stage of clarification have been classified in 5 categories of items; they split rather differently according to the teams.

Item "ethics", 14 verbatims (lowest priorities): confidential aspect and data security, therapist/patient relation to be protected, difficult relation of some therapists with medical informatics.

Table 1.

Nr Team	Doctors			Physiotherapists			Nurses		
	Incoded sub-contacts	Performed acts	**Relation contacts / acts**	Incoded sub-contacts	Performed acts	**Relation contacts / acts**	Incoded sub-contacts	Performed acts	**Relation contacts / acts**
7	11408	5638	**2.02**	635	1252	**0.51**	197	626	**0.31**
REF1	10507	17595	**0.60**	2205	6182	**0.36**	0	4414	**0.00**
REF2	5534	3020	**1.83**	5	582	**0.01**	1	178	**0.01**
REF3	10890	8299	**1.31**	4313	3251	**1.33**	731	1515	**0.48**
REF4	13238	4938	**2.68**	620	1662	**0.37**	1534	1826	**0.84**
Okkes			**1.1 to 1.7**						

Item "training", 21 verbatims (average priority): fundamental training to data processing, forming to logical reasoning (supposed or real) of computerized records, practical organization of those formings: pleasant, continuous, on the spot.

Item "search for sense", 49 verbatims (rank of priority in the high average): local output, statistics, and desire for using them in plans aiming at increasing quality of care; possible data sharing, essentially to compare with other practitioners or for common actions; specific forming to reach these objectives; a greater motivation: exchanges with happy users, explanation of the meaning of epidemiology, of public health.

Item "practice", 72 verbatims (average to high priority). Half of it had to do with the software improvement. The other half concerned solutions linked to the internal organization or to the time spent to the use of computers (training, data recording).

Item "interdisciplinarity", 21 verbatims (high priority): a better coordination between professional sectors, work where everyone feels supported by a collective effort, carrying out of projects.

3. Discussion

Data collection in a regional epidemiological aim is a short range objective accessible to some teams. Its quality must still be validated.

A local use of the consultation data in the aim of quality of care improvement should be generalized. The practical solutions imagined by the teams we met may constitute the basis of a support action program.

3.1. Results of the Intervention

The quantitative measures on the databases of the visited teams have confirmed the slight use of EMR. Three teams on eight however have made the first step towards a computerization of their data and this on various stages; an interdisciplinary use seems possible.

Those teams forms a rather heterogeneous unity as for the solutions they viewed, the priority stage they gave them. Moreover, this little sample only included teams that were very motivated by computerization. The collected results must be considered as a qualitative reflection of the blockings. The measure of quantitative indicators in the reference teams showed differences in behaviour between practitioners: the use rates of the EMR when consulting and the effective interdisciplinary use are rather varying.

3.1.1. The Practical Side

The very great number of requests viewing the software improvement conveys a certain exasperation of the users. The fear of loosing time because of data processing is very present, specially during the consultation and, to a lesser degree, in forming.

The teams have identified their forming needs, first in basic informatics, then in the logic of medical informatics. The wish of forming to exploit the data strengthen the need of a structured and codified information. The reluctance of using classifications, found in my experience [3, 8] as in literature [9], hasn't been expressed any more in the nominal groups.

3.1.2. Motivation and Interdisciplinarity

Three points mark the original feature of Belgian Medical Houses. There is a strong demand to see the outcome to learn things about the served patients or about the team organization. This strengthens the importance of the local loop for the quality of collected data [2].

The internal organization of the teams has been recognized as one of the brakes. The self administrative way of working can raise the number of responsible persons of being convinced of the validity of changes [10].

The wish of a local data sharing with a software oriented towards the pure medical logics generates frustrations by the paramedical personal. In those self-managed interdisciplinary teams, what is at stake is as important as having a common language and objectives [11] as those of the liberal networks of home-coordinated care [12]. The data sharing clashes with the differences between the members: facing the technique, facing motivation, facing available time.

3.1.3. Ethics

As far as the security of the data is concerned, half of the teams seems to have no worry, and that is disturbing. The flaws in security are potentially more important in a bigger network [13]. The question of data transfer for an epidemiological use has not been evoked. The place given to the computer in the relationship with the patient doesn't take an important place in the present worries, but most of the teams are not confronted with this problem.

3.2. Action Proposals to be Developed

If the objectives are partly shared, the needs of the teams can, at a given moment, clearly differ. The ideal is to create conditions of a distinctive accompaniment in a whole movement.

An audit of the situation of each team before computerization would be useful: knowledge, attitudes and practices of the members, equipment, pursued objectives, time of bringing it to play and available funding. The planning of changes can be inspired by existing programs [14], and the logical follow-up consists in giving that allows solving of identified problems.

The practitioners expressed the need of having a tool easy to use, that doesn't make them lose time and that has respect for their specificity of work and organization (interdisciplinary and self-managed teams), or it will create a deep-seated allergy to machines [15]. It must propose typical interfaces for paramedical professions, structured around the central point of record: the patient's list of episodes. To reach the aim, the users must be more closely associated to the different phases of development.

The practitioners are willing to computerize if they get immediate advantages (knowledge of their patients and their team operating). In spite of a software that is often considered as unapproachable, some teams already use the EMR and treat data. A widely spread information must make it possible to show the obtained results and their impact on practice, as the met difficulties.

The users expressed the need of an external support, under the form of adapted training and supervision for the data management. The forming persons must get closer to their needs and demands, meet them on their workplace. The failure met by the participants, reluctant to accept "glorious" predictions of a radiant future, can be discussed [16, 17].

A support structure has to be made operational, so that it will be possible to propose wholes of requests which give answers to the most frequent questions. If necessary, this structure should also be able to process the data and advise the pertinence of collecting this or that parameter or indicator. The British and Dutch efforts which have been accepted in the 80s in collaboration with the professional organizations [18, 19, 20] have ended-up in large scale projects which favour the data collection in primary care and its feed-back towards the practitioners [21, 22]. The Belgian situation is less favourable, but is developing at the moment in the right direction [23, 24, 25].

The basic principles of computerized data security are different from those which are applicable to a room with files on a note trolley [26]. A piece of information about security strategies, procedures and official requirements is all the more essential since the demand is weak.

4. Conclusion

The practitioners are willing to improve the quality of care through self evaluation or projects. Specific tools and training have to be developed and proposed. Professional organizations and authorities have a leading part in developing this quality improvement.

References

[1] Lamberts H, Mennerat F, Okkes I. Dossier de patient structure en épisodes et analyse des données en médecine générale 1. La réalité aux Pays-Bas. In Venot A, Falcoff H. L'Informatisation du Cabinet Médical du Futur, Volume 11. Paris, Springer-Verlag France,1999.

[2] Lagasse R, Desmet M, Jamoulle M, et al. European situation of the routine data collection and their utilisation for health monitoring. Euro-Med-Data. Final report. Bruxelles:Ecole de santé publique, Université libre de Bruxelles. Déc. 2001.

[3] Prévost M, Della Giustina V, Gosselain Y, et al. Gestion de l'information dans les pratiques de soins intégrés. Santé conjuguée 2002.19:5-11.

[4] Vanmeerbeek M, Berquin E. Le recueil systématique de données dans le dossier médical informatisé comme outil d'aide à la prise en charge du patient diabétique. Communication au Colloque des Maisons médicales. Blankenberghe. Mai 2004.

[5] Delbecq AL, Van de Ven AH. A group process model for problem identification and program planning. Journal of Applied Behavioral Sciences, 1975.7:466-480.

[6] Pineault R, Daveluy C. La planification de la santé. Concepts, méthodes, stratégies. Montréal:Les Editions Agence d'Arc,1986:236-240.

[7] Okkes IM et al. The role of family practice in different health care systems: a comparison of reasons for encounter, diagnoses, and interventions in primary care populations in the Netherlands, Japan, Poland, and the United States. J Fam Pract. 2002.51(Jan):72-3.

[8] Havelange C. La trace, construction d'un récit. Santé conjuguée, 2002.19:12-13. Transcription de V. Della Giustina.

[9] de Lusignan S, Wells SE, Hague NJ, Thiru K. Managers see the problems associated with coding clinical data as a technical issue whilst clinicians also see cultural barriers. Methods Inf Med., 2003.42(4):416-22.

[10] Ladavid C. Le système « autogestionnaire » en maisons médicales : analyse de cas. Santé conjuguée, 2004.28(avril):13.

[11] Recommandations pour la tenue du dossier de soins infirmiers du malade à domicile. Perspectives d'avenir et informatisation. ANAES, guides méthodologiques, juin 1997.

[12] Latignies O, Brohée A, Lamy D, et al. Le projet CRISNET, outil open source pour le dossier médical partagé en réseau. Communication au sixième atelier du CISP-Club. Mons, Belgique, 24-26 octobre 2003.

[13] Benson T. Why general practitioners use computers and hospital doctors do not-Part 2: scalability. BMJ, 2002.325:1090-1093.

[14] Carrupt M. Nouvelles technologies : conditions de réussite d'implantation dans le secteur de la santé. http://www.cmic.ch/formation/projet_informatique.pdf p.5-9 consulted 08/08/2004.

[15] Asimov I. Les cavernes d'acier, Hachette, 1956.

[16] Sittig Dean F et al. Techniques for Identifying the Applicability of New Information. Management Technologies in the Clinical Setting:An Example Focusing on Handheld Computers. Proc AMIA Symp. 2000:804-8.

[17] Stavri PZ, Ash JS. Does failure breed success : narrative analysis of stories about computerized provider order entry. Int J Med Inf., 2003.72(1-3):9-15.

[18] Benson T. Why general practitioners use computers and hospital doctors do not-Part 1: incentives. BMJ, 2002.325:1086-1089.

[19] Royal College of General Practitioners. General practice computerisation. London: RCGP, 2000:RCGP information sheet October 2000 No7.

[20] van der Lei J, Duisterhout JS, Westerhof HP, et al. The introduction of computer-based patient records in The Netherlands. Ann Intern Med., 1993.15;119(10):1036-41.
[21] Primis. Data quality analysis service. The University of Nottingham. http://www.primis.nottingham.ac.uk/pages/Data_Quality_Analysis.asp?om=m2 consulted 02/09/2004.
[22] http://www.linh.nl/ consulted 08/10/2004.
[23] Groupe de travail EMDMI. Dossier médical informatisé. Bruxelles:SPF Santé publique, Sécurité de la Chaîne alimentaire et Environnement, 2003.
[24] Declerck E. ResoPrim, réseau expérimental en soins de santé primaires. Bruxelles:document public du SPF de Programmation de la Politique Scientifique 9/12/03.
[25] Vandenberghe H, Bastiaens H, Jonckheer P et al. Amélioration de la qualité en médecine générale sur base d'enregistrements de données de consultation: diabète de type 2 et hypertension artérielle - Rapport final. Bruxelles:Institut Scientifique de la Santé Publique, juin 2003:IPH/EPI REPORTS N° 2003 – 09.
[26] Anderson R. NHS-wide networking and patient confidentiality. BMJ, 1995.311:5-6 Editorials.

Health Continuum and Data Exchange in Belgium and in the Netherlands
Francis H. Roger France et al. (Eds.)
IOS Press, 2004

PropeR and Archetypes

Helma VAN DER LINDEN, Huibert TANGE and Jan TALMON
University Maastricht, Medical Informatics
POBOX 616, 6200 MD Maastricht, The Netherlands

Abstract. The PropeR project studies a genric combination of an electronic health record (EHR) and decision support software (DSS). This study comprises different medical domains. GOAL – develop a distributed EHR system that is flexible enough to be used in different domains without major modifications. METHODS – use of standards and standardized specification and available open source components to develop an EHR system that meets the goals. RESULT – PropeRWeb is a generic webbased EHR system that is flexible enough to easily accommodate different domains. DISCUSSION – discussion of some of the problems encountered in the development of the EHR system.

Keywords. Computerized Medical Records Systems, Systems Integration, Software Design, standards, components, open source

Introduction

The PropeR project [1] started in 2000 to study the combination of decision support software (DSS) and an EHR in two settings. The first setting is the domain of stroke patients receiving rehabilitation in their home environment by a multidisciplinary team of primary care therapists [2]. The second setting is the protocol based treatment of AML (Acute Myeloid Leukemia) patients in the hematology department of the Maastricht Academic Hospital. This article focuses on the development of the EHR system.

1. Goals

The first goal in the project was identified as the development of an EHR system that would meet the needs of the primary care team, but at the same time would be flexible enough to be adjusted for the other subproject without major adjustments. This EHR system had to meet the following requirements:

- accommodate data from multiple disciplines;
- extendable to connect to a decision support (DSS) component;
- integrate data from various data sources;
- available at various locations;
- standards-compliant;
- allow a change of domain without major modifications;
- be robust enough to last beyond the scope of the project.

2. Methods

Research showed that, at the time, there was no system that would meet all our requirements. We therefore decided to build our own. We focused on the use of the OMG HDTF[1] specifications Person Identification Specification (PIDS) and Clinical Observation Access Specification (COAS) [3, 4] and the use of open source components to speed up the development process, while still allowing the extension of the software for the necessary connection to the DSS component.

The OMG HDTF specifications provide a generic interface to various servers. This simplifies the implementation of integrating various data sources. By separating patient demographic information in PIDS servers and medical data in COAS servers, not only the privacy of the patient is enhanced, but the medical data is also automatically anonymized, which makes them more readily available for research. The OpenEMed implementation of PIDS and COAS is generally recognized as reference implementation of the OMG HDTF specifications.

To further standardize the data modeling we used the archetype specification of the OpenEHR project [5, 6]. Archetypes are machine readable definition of medical concepts, roughly equivalent to HL7 templates. By constructing archetypes from generic building blocks, which can in turn be stored in a generic database, it is possible to delegate the definition of medical concepts in archetypes to medical specialists. The generic software for handling archetypes can then be built by software specialists. Development of archetypes and software can then be done in different paces. This principle can be identified as a “Separation of Disciplines”.

Study of COAS and archetypes learned that the two specifications are complementary: where COAS defines structure, archetypes define content.

The architecture of the system is service-based. Three layers can be recognized:

- A back-end containing the PIDS servers and COAS servers with their respective databases,
- A middle layer containing the kernel and the archetype definitions and
- A presentation layer handling the user interaction.

3. Results

The resulting system, named PropeRWeb, is a webbased system written in Java. Figure 1 shows a schematic view of the system.
The OpenEMed [7] PIDS and COAS servers are used as data services. The middleware is currently implemented using the open source OpenORB, which is CORBA-based.

The Cocoon Framework [8] is used for presentation and user interaction. The client side of the system consists of nothing more than a web browser. A recent version of the browser is requested to allow proper handling of the javascripts that are used to improve user friendliness.

The kernel (grey in Figure 1) was developed in-house. It handles the connections to the PIDS and COAS servers and manipulates the archetype definitions to either convert them to a Cocoon-compliant structure for user interaction or a PIDS or COAS-compliant structure for storage or querying and retrieval. There are two separate repositories for archetypes and for forms. A PropeRWeb form is defined as a container for one or more related archetypes. It is complemented with screen representations for review and editing of the information in the archetypes. As figure 1 shows both archetype definitions and form definitions are stored outside the kernel. They are implemented as XML documents. It is therefore pos-

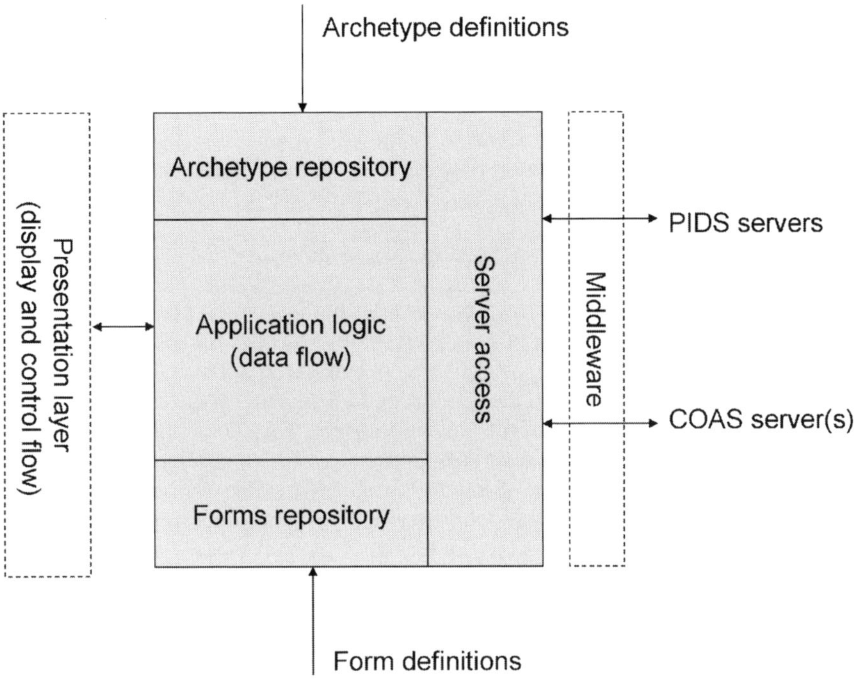

Figure 1. Schematic view of PropeRWeb, with the kernel (in grey) in more detail.

sible to replace the archetype and form definitions of one domain with those of a completely different domain with hardly any modifications to the software. Although not shown in Figure 1, the screen definitions are also stored as external documents which also allows for easy modification of the user interface.

The system was tested on various operating systems such as Windows 2000, Windows XP, Linux in various flavours and Mac OS X. In all situations the system worked as expected and proved to be stable.

4. Discussion

The development of an EHR system based on standards and components, preferably using existing open source, turned out to be more complex than expected:

- The OMG HDTF specifications PIDS and COAS have a steep learning curve and it takes a considerable amount of time to appreciate the full implication of the specifications.
- The archetype specification is very elaborately documented but is also an elaborate specification that could not be readily implemented in the course of the project.
- Another issue we came across when defining archetypes was the level of granularity of the concepts to be defined.
- We used the components of the open source projects OpenEMed and OpenORB. They proved to be of excellent quality and the lack of extensive documentation was compensated by the adequate responses from the communities. Still, since both are complex

projects implementation required quite some time to study and get familiar with the features and the concepts.

- Using existing software, as opposed to tailor-made software, means that the provided functionality might not fully cover the requirements. This was true for OpenEMed.
- At first the presentation layer was developed with Java Server Pages (JSPs). As development progressed the distinction between the presentation layer and the kernel disappeared.

In the current version, these issues are addressed as follows:

- We simplified the implementation of archetypes to the simplest possible definition. This reduced the time necessary to fully implement all aspect of the archetype specification as well as remove some of the complexity that could lead to errors.
- This simplification also lead to the conclusion to define archetypes at the lowest level of granularity possible, i.e. that of the medical concept. This would also promote the reuse of identical medical concepts in various forms.
- When the first implementation using JSPs was not flexible enough for the increasing complexity of the PropeRWeb system, a major rewrite was necessary. Rather than using the same techniques, we decided to use Cocoon which provided a much richer presentation framework than we could ever have built in a short time, yet allowed to scale it down to a simple application.
- Both OpenEMed and Cocoon are used in various other projects, which contributes to the generic nature of the software. Where possible we redesigned the necessary functionality to use the software of both projects with as few modifications as possible. For OpenEMed we proposed an extension we needed. The Cocoon community itself added code that would make the integration of the PropeRWeb kernel easier.

5. Lessons Learned

Building an EHR system based on standard and components is not as straight forward as one would assume. From the development of the PropeRWeb we learned:

- Although specifications are elaborate and well documented, actual implementation in software reveals the ambiguities and problems.
- Designing software, especially in a research setting, cannot avoid running into unforeseen problems during implementation. Rather than trying to fix the problems with the least possible change in design and/or code, a complete rewrite using different techniques often results in a much better quality and flexibility of the software and justifies the learning curve and the extra time necessary to get acquainted with the new techniques.
- Software for healthcare is very specific and more complex than a counterpart in another domain. It is therefore not possible to simply assume that time and effort required to develop e.g. a banking application is equal to developing a similar application for healthcare.
- Using complex open source projects such as OpenEMed and Cocoon requires either extensive documentation or an active community. If one or both are present all the advantages usually stated in a discussion on open source are true. If both lack, it depends on the perceived quality of the software and the ability of the user to interpret the source code, whether there is an advantage.

6. Test Plan

Although the first version of PropeRWeb proved to be stable on multiple platforms, we intend to repeat this test with the Cocoon version. Simultaneously the flexibility will be tested by defining a different set of definitions for the AML domain. Finally the functionality of the software will be tested by both primary care users and the team at the hematology department.

Endnotes

[1] The OMG HDTF is the Object Management Group's Healthcare Domain Taskforce. The OMG is an international, open membership, not-for-profit consortium that produces and maintains computer industry specifications for interoperable enterprise applications (http://www.omg.org). Virtually all large companies in the computer industry are members.

References

[1] H. van der Linden, G. Boers, H. Tange, J. Talmon, A. Hasman, PropeR: a multidisciplinary EPR system, Int J Med Inform 70 (2003) 149-160.

[2] anonymous, Transmuraal Zorgmodel CVA Regio Heuvelland (in Dutch), Synchron, Heerlen april 1996.

[3] anonymous, Person Identification Service (PIDS) Specification, Version 1.1, http://cgi.omg.org/docs/formal/01-04-04.pdf, 2001, Last accessed: 2004/09/14.

[4] anonymous, Clinical Observations Access Service Specification, Version 1.0, http://cgi.omg.org/docs/formal/01-04-06.pdf, 2001, Last accessed: 2004/09/14.

[5] anonymous, OpenEHR, http://www.openehr.org, Last accessed: 2004/09/14.

[6] T. Beale, Archetypes Constraint-based Domain Models for Future-proof Information Systems, Revision 2.2.1, http://www.deepthought.com.au/it/archetypes/archetypes.pdf, 2001, Last accessed: 2004/09/14.

[7] anonymous, OpenEMed, http://www.openemed.org, Last accessed: 2004/09/14.

[8] anonymous, The Apache Cocoon Framework, http://cocoon.apache.org, Last accessed: 2004/09/14.

Contact address

H. van der Linden
Universiteit Maastricht
POBox 616
6200 MD Maastricht
The Netherlands
Email: h.vanderlinden@mi.unimaas.nl

Health Continuum and Data Exchange in Belgium and in the Netherlands
Francis H. Roger France et al. (Eds.)
IOS Press, 2004

Incorporating Evaluation into the Design of a Decision-Support System

Stefan VISSCHER, Karin SCHURINK and Marc BONTEN
Department of Internal Medicine and Infectious Diseases
University Medical Centre Utrecht
{S.Visscher, K.Schurink, M.J.M.Bonten}@azu.nl

Peter LUCAS
Institute for Computing and Information Sciences
Radboud University Nijmegen
peterl@cs.ru.nl

Jeroen VAN WOLFFELAAR and Peter VAN DE WERKEN
Institute of Information and Computing Sciences
Utrecht University
{jjawolff, pwerken}@cs.uu.nl

Abstract. Medical decision support systems will only be accepted by the medical community if properly evaluated. However, little attention has been given in the scientific literature to the topic of how to incorporate evaluation issues into the design of a decision-support system. In this paper, we describe work in developing a decision-support system that is intended to support the management (diagnosis and treatment selection) of ventilator-associated pneumonia in patients. From the beginning of the development of this system, we have taken care to incorporate evaluation issues into the design of the system. In the paper, we analyse the problems that need be taken into account when evaluating a system. Next, we describe the consequences for the functionality of the system.

Keywords. Decision-Support System, Decision Theory, Bayesian Network, Evaluation Biases, Ventilator-Associated Pneumonia, Antibiotics, Intensive Care Unit

Introduction

The management, i.e. the diagnosis and the selection of optimal treatment, of disorders in critical care is a challenging task, as patients are usually severely ill and often have a number of concomitant disorders; thus if treatment is delayed this may be the cause of death of a patient. Diagnosing a disorder is in particular difficult if there are few signs and symptoms that are typical for the disorder and if a disorder does not occur very frequently. Furthermore, selecting optimal treatment is difficult as there is normally no time to wait with instilling treatment until the results of laboratory tests become available. This is, for example, the situation with ventilator-associated pneumonia, or VAP for short. VAP is a form of pneumonia that occurs in patients whom are mechanically ventilated in critical care units, with signs and symptoms, such as high body temperature and high numbers of white blood cells (leukocytosis) that are shared by many other disorders critically ill patients may have. Hence, diagnosing, and therefore also treating, VAP is difficult. This has implications for the management of patients with VAP, as it is quite unlikely that Intensive Care Unit (ICU) doctors are able to identify this disorder reliably, and prescribe optimal treatment. It is therefore believed my many clinical experts in the field of VAP that ICU doctors need some form of decision support.

In this paper we describe our work in the design of an architecture for a decision-support system (DSS) that allows evaluating the efficacy of use of the system in a critical-care environment. It is argued that in developing a DSS for clinical use, more attention should be given to evaluation issues than currently is the case. However, the wish to evaluate a DSS has also consequences for its user interface and organisation. In this paper we relate general considerations found in the literature on evaluation to an actual architecture of a DSS.

The structure of the paper is as follows. In the following section, previous research in computer-based clinical decision support is described. In Section 3, the problem of the management of VAP is described and the model that underlies our DSS is summarised in Section 4. In Section 5, we analyse considerations with respect to evaluation for the architecture of the DSS. The resulting architecture is subsequently described in Section 6. The paper is rounded off by some conclusions.

1. Previous Research

Over the last decades, much progress has been made in diagnosing and treating disorders in patients. The medical community itself has introduced clinical guidelines as a vehicle of quality improvement and control, and an increasing number of clinical guidelines have become available. Modern clinical guidelines are evidence-based, i.e. based on results reported in the scientific literature, and are meant to support clinicians in their decision-making process. These clinical guidelines may contain cost components, organisational aspects and aspects for implementation. The main purpose of a clinical guideline is to provide a standard that allows for all physicians to generalise the management of patients with a specific disorder or illness and to reduce variation between physicians [2]. However, very few physicians use a guideline when it is available on paper only. Computerising these clinical guidelines eases their use, but most guidelines are designed with use on paper in mind, and it is therefore not straightforward to convert them into executable form.

An alternative to quality improvement of clinical care is being offered by DSSs. In contrast to medical guidelines, medical DSSs are normally computer-based from the start and thinking about the design of such systems involves taking into account how computer-based systems can best offer support to the clinical user. These computer systems contain medical knowledge provided by medical specialists, but can, of course, also be evidence-based as modern guidelines. By helping physicians in their management process, a decision-support system aims to enhance patient outcomes.

There are many ways in which a DSS can be constructed. As the management of patients with a disorder involves uncertainty, due to the fact that the state of the patient is incompletely known, and tradeoffs between pros and cons of various treatment modalities, we think that Bayesian networks combined with decision theory offers the most suitable basis for such systems [3].

2. The Problem: Incorporating Evaluation into the Design of a DSS

Most medical DSSs are designed and developed taking only into account their final use. However, it has been stated again and again that for DSS to be accepted by the clinical community it is essential that they are properly evaluated. This will have implications for the functionality and organisation of a DSS. For example, to obtain faithful evaluation results it is necessary that a DSS does not influence the decisions made by a clinician. Clearly, this requirement contradicts the final use of a medical DSS, which is expected to support clinical decision making, and thus to improve and change the clinician's decisions. The question, therefore, arises to what extent evaluation requirements are compatible with the intension to produce a final working system, and to which extent incorporated evaluation facilities restrict use of the final system. These questions are being addressed in this paper for the specific system we developed for the management of VAP.

3. A DSS for VAP: its Underlying Bayesian-Network and Decision-Theoretic Model

The DSS for the management of VAP we developed is based on a Bayesian network and also incorporates a decision-theoretic part to make treatment choices. We will only provide a brief summary here; a more detailed description of the Bayesian network and decision-theoretic model, including a motivation for their structure and content, is given in Ref. [7].

A Bayesian network consists of two parts: a qualitative part, i.e. the structure of the network including all relations between the variables, and a quantitative part, i.e. conditional probabilities $P(X \mid pa(X))$ for each variable X associated with a vertex V, where pa(X) stands for the set of variables associated with the parents of V. The model for the management of VAP consists of a diagnostic part and a prognostic part. The structure of the diagnostic part is concerned with the diagnosis of VAP, based on the patient's clinical signs, the duration of stay in the hospital and whether or not the patient is mechanically ventilated. To be able to identify the bacteria, which may have been the cause of the pneumonia, the process of bacterial colonisation as taking place in the ICU has also been modelled. For the construction of the quantitative part, the infectious-disease expert had to estimate all conditional probabilities. The prognostic part of the Bayesian network is intended to provide information about the most effective combination of antibiotics, i.e. it is used to determine optimal coverage for VAP. As determining the optimal treatment uses decision theory; the VAP expert was asked to provide utilities for all sensible combinations of antibiotics, taking into account presence and absence of VAP, side effects, financial costs and antimicrobial spectrum.

The global structure of the resulting Bayesian-network model is shown in Figure 1.

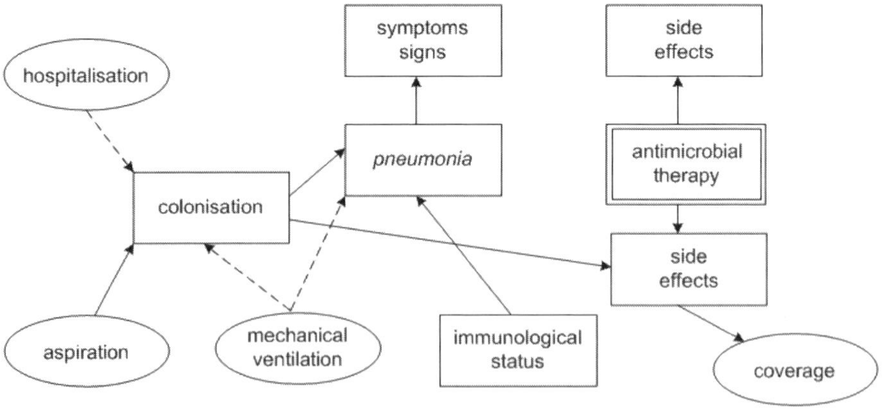

Figure 1. Global structure of the Bayesian-network model for VAP; single-lined boxes stand for sets of variables, and antimicrobial therapy is the decision variable.

4. Design of an Evaluation Study of the DSS for VAP

There are a number of issues that must be taken into account when evaluating a DSS. These issues are described here. We also describe how a resulting system can be evaluated. Subsequently in Section 6 the consequences for the architecture and functionality of the DSS are discussed in detail.

4.1. Evaluation Biases

When using a DSS in a particular user environment, such as the management of a disorder in an ICU, evaluation results may not faithfully reflect the reality due to unknown systematic effects. These confounding effects, or biases, have to be taken into account before designing an evaluation study. Known types of biases include [1]:

- The *volunteer effect*: doctors who volunteer to use the system perform better than others. A possible explanation for this effect is that a volunteer is probably more willing to use the system than someone who is not volunteering;
- The *assessment bias*: knowledge of gold standard or system output may influence the user's decisions. Since there is no real gold standard for the management of VAP, this does not apply. However, when taken into account the system's output, the judgement of a doctor might be influenced by it.
- The *Hawthorne effect*: clinical performance improves if clinicians know they are being studied.
- The *checklist effect*: performance improves if clinicians use a checklist. When using a checklist, a clinician is reminded of the factors that are considered relevant in, for example, diagnosing a certain disorder. This may cause improvement in clinical performance.

Clearly, when evaluating a DSS these biases cannot be ignored, but should be addressed somehow. We will do so in the following.

4.2. Design of the Study

Considering the discussed evaluation biases, we designed the evaluation study for the system as follows. As the Hawthorn effect is difficult to avoid, we will ask *all* ICU doctors to use the decision-support system. By doing so, we make the assumption that all doctors behave like the employees in the Hawthorne factory [8]. Thus, in case usage of our DSS causes a change in diagnostic behaviour, we in a way take into account this bias, as it has been incorporated in all performance measurements. We eliminate the volunteer effect: in this study, as every ICU doctor is expected to use the system when is not particularly reluctant to use the system. As the three ICUs of the University Medical Centre Utrecht that act as our study environment use an electronic patients record system, the doctors are already used to the deployment of a computer-based system in the patient-care process. By making sure that the system does not give an advice concerning a patient before having asked the doctor to enter his or her expert opinion, the possibility that the doctor's original opinion is influenced by the system's output is eliminated.

5. Resulting DSS for VAP

The decision-support system that is described in this paper is intended to be operating within the ICUs of the University Medical Centre Utrecht. Building the system, we had to take the evaluation biases, described in the previous section, into account. As such, it is necessary that the system is integrated with the clinical information system that is used in the ICUs. This system is a full-fletched system that functions as an electronic patient records system (EPR). As no paper patient records are used any more within the three ICUs deploying the EPR, this system contains a wealth of patient information which can be exploited for decision-support purposes.

5.1. Components of the System

The front-end of the DSS consists of a graphical user interface (GUI) with pop-up menus, tables and some graphics, allowing clinicians to enter patient data and to inspect patient data, mostly in textual form, but sometimes – for certain laboratory data – in graphical form, as a time plot. The back-end is a relational database management system, which is linked to the EPR system's relational database system. This not only offers modern facility for secure data storage, updating and retrieval, but also a Structured Query Language (SQL) interface, allowing external systems access to the data.

It was decided to develop a separate user-interface for the decision-support system in particular because this makes separate development possible. We used modern distributed information system technology, in our case Hypertext Preprocessor (PHP). PHP is a server-side HTML-embedded cross-platform scripting language, which allows one to generate content of HTML pages dynamically.

PHP is actually used as the language to link various parts of the system together. The majority of the functionality of the system is offered by a commercially available Bayesian-network and decision-network package, which is used in our project to implement the inference engine for the decision-support system. This part of the system processes patient data, and offers various types of advice based on the results computed after instantiating the Bayesian network model of VAP with the patient data. This advice is presented to the user.

The final components for the system are an HTTP server, and a Web browser. The HTTP server that is used in the project is Apache. The Web browser acts as the user interface to the decision-support system.

The architecture of the system is visualised in Figure 2.

5.2. Added Facilities for Evaluation

For every patient who is mechanically ventilated, the doctor is asked for his or her expert opinion. When a VAP is concerned, also the prescribed antibiotic or combination of antibi-

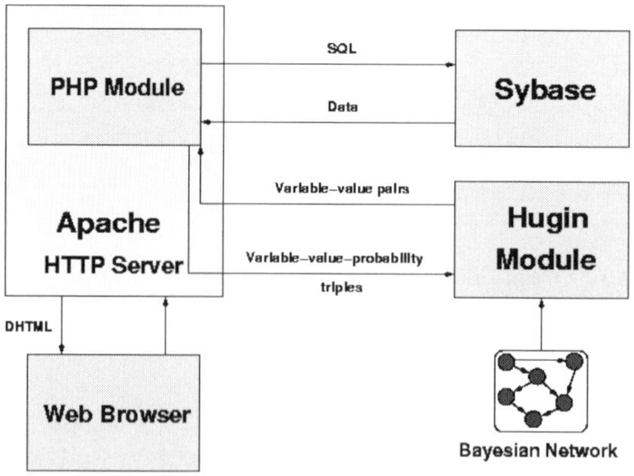

Figure 2. Global architecture of the system.

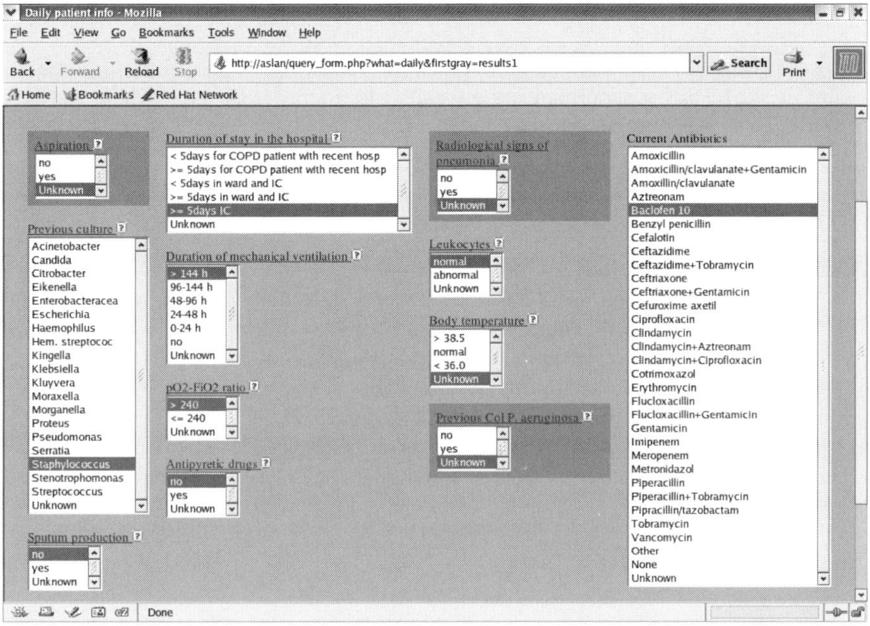

Figure 3. A screenshot of a form that is part of the DSS representing symptoms of the patient.

otics is filled in, including the motivation for this choice. Following this, a form is shown, representing the patient's clinical details. See Figure 3 for a screenshot of this form. These values are pre-selected from the clinical database and, when the doctor disagrees, he or she can change them. This form, or checklist, might be a confounding factor. Unfortunately, measuring or expressing this effect is difficult, if not impossible. But since all physicians are expected to fill in the checklist, measurement of the effect is not necessary. After the physician has filled in the checklist, a management advice is presented to the user *at random*, i.e. on average in 50% of the consultations of the system an advice is obtained and in 50% of cases, no advice is being offered. The advice, if being offered, includes the likelihood for the patient of having VAP and the optimal treatment for possible colonisation of the respiratory tract. By doing so, we are able to compare the two groups of doctors who were or were not presented with an advice. Only when the system's advice is presented, the doctor is asked again whether he or she suspects the patient having pneumonia, and which therapy, i.e. combination of antibiotics, he or she wishes to prescribe, taking into account the system's advice. In this way, we are able to see if the physician changed his or her judgement after the presented advice. One possibility is that the physician has become more aware of some important symptoms of the patient, so that he or she revised the earlier judgement. Another possibility is that the physician did not change his or her decision after the system's output, simply due to ignoring the advice or because filling in the symptoms did not change the physician's view regarding the patient. From this we can draw conclusions concerning the influence of the system's advice on the physician's judgement.

6. Conclusions

Medical decision-support systems are meant to assist clinicians in the difficult process of medical management. As was argued, the availability of medical decision support is even more crucial in a critical care environment, as mistakes made by doctors usually have drastic consequences for the patient. However, certainly in critical care environments doctors are reluctant to use DSS that have not been evaluated clinically. We have, therefore, taking an actual DSS that supports the management of VAP as an example, developed a medical DSS environment that incorporates facilities for clinical evaluation. The reasons for including these facilities were motivated. We believe that more attention should be given to evaluation issues, when developing medical DSSs than has been done so far. When these evaluation issues are incorporated into the design of a decision-support system, it is possible to perform a reliable evaluation of such system by its users even when using it in a real-life setting.

References

[1] Friedman, C. & Wyatt, J. (1997). Evaluation methods in medical informatics. Springer-Verlag, New York. ("Computers & Medicine" series.) ISBN 0-387-94228-9.

[2] Kocher MS, Mandiga R, Murphy JM, Goldmann D, Harper M, Sundel R, Ecklund K, Kasser JR. A clinical practice guideline for treatment of septic arthritis in children. *The Journal of Bone and Joint Surgery (American)* 2003; 85: 994–999.

[3] Lucas PJF, Boot H, Taal BG. Computer-based decision support in the management of primary gastric non-Hodgkin lymphoma. *Methods of Information in Medicine*, 37:206 – 219, 1998.

[4] Bonten MJM, Kollef MH, Hall JB. Risk factors for ventilator-associated pneumonia: from epidemiology to patient management. *Clinical Infectious Diseases* 2004; 38(8): 1141-9.

[5] Bonten MJM, Bergmans CJJ, Ambergen AW, De Leeuw PW, Van der Geest S, Stobberingh EE, Gaillard CA. Factors for pneumonia and colonization of respiratory tract and stomach in mechanically-ventilated ICU patients. *Am J Respir Crit Care Med* 1996; 154: 1339–1346.

[6] Lucas PJF, Van der Gaag LC. *Principles of Expert Systems*. Wokingham: Addison-Wesley, 1991.

[7] Lucas PJF, de Bruijn NC, Schurink CAM, Hoepelman IM. A Probabilistic and decision-theoretic approach to the management of infectious disease at the ICU. *Artificial Intelligence in Medicine* 2000; 19(3): 251–279.

[8] Mayo E. (1933) *The human problems of an industrial civilization* (New York: MacMillan) ch.3.

[9] Berner ES, Maisiak RS, Cobbs GC, Taunton DO. Effects of a Decision Support System on Physicians' Diagnostic Perfomance. *Journal of the American Medical Informatics Association* 1999; 6: 420–427.

Contact information:

Drs. Stefan Visscher (S.Visscher@azu.nl)
University Medical Centre Utrecht
Department of Internal Medicine and Infectious Diseases
Huispostnr. F.02.126
Heidelberglaan 100
3584CX Utrecht

Health Continuum and Data Exchange in Belgium and in the Netherlands
Francis H. Roger France et al. (Eds.)
IOS Press, 2004

Introduction of an Operating Room Information Management System Improved Overall Operating Room Efficiency

Cathy DE DEYNE and René HEYLEN
Dept of Anesthesia and Critical Care Medicine
Ziekenhuis Oost-Limburg ZOL – Genk (Belgium)

Abstract. Operating Room (OR) information systems should manage the OR time, assigned to every surgeon, thereby minimizing the sum of costs of unused OR time and minimizing the costs of elective cases performed outside normal allocated OR time (excess OR-time). The aim of this paper is to illustrate how the introduction of an OR information system influenced daily OR activity performance.

Since January 2001, we introduced an OR information system with a visual, airport-like, screen as central part, displaying all scheduled OR activity linked in real-time activity with all OR theatres. For the aim of this paper, we compared all data of OR activity for elective abdominal surgery (EAS) for the first half of 2000 compared to the first half of 2001, after the introduction of our information system.

In 2000, 764 elective cases were performed, compared to 815 cases in 2001. For both periods, the total OR time allocated to EAS for this 6 months period was 805 h. For 2000, the total duration of OR activity for EAS was 1044h50min (implicating 239h50min over-time), compared to 1127h35min (implicating 322h35min over-time) for 2001. For 2000, we recorded 147h20min excess time (=exceeding the time limits of OR activity and inducing extra costs) and 46h45min unused OR time. For 2001, we recorded 123h04min excess time and 35h21min unused time.

In conclusion, in 2001 we recorded an increase in total OR activity for elective abdominal surgery by 7% in number of procedures and by 8% in total duration. However, in 2001 we recorded a decrease in excess time by 16% (123h04min vs 147h20min), which was for a large part due to a 23% decrease in unused OR time in 2001 compared to 2000 (35h21min vs 46h45min). Therefore, the introduction of an OR information system, with a real-time visual display of ongoing OR activity, resulted in a increased performance of OR activity, with more OR procedures performed despite less excess time and less extra costs.

Keywords. Operating Room, Information Management System, Operating Room Efficiency

Introduction

Operating room (OR) activity plays an important and sometimes pivotal role in the financial budget of the total hospital activity [1]. Therefore, it is of utmost importance to acquire an accurate and up-dated information on the structure of overall OR activity costs. A lot of published data analyzed the exact structure of these total OR activity costs. They revealed that not the direct costs (such as medication, material, etc…) but the indirect costs take the largest part of the total OR budget. These indirect costs contain all fixed (administrative support, buildings, technical support) and semivariable (nursing staff) costs and are for most of them not directly related to the incurred number of OR procedures [2,3]. Therefore, not the number of OR procedures, but the efficient use of OR time is the major factor of total OR activity costs. Every minute of OR time used or un-used is the main determinator, as every minute of maximally staffed OR time costs a lot of money, especially if there is no financial return in case no OR procedure is performed. Therefore, every available minute of OR time should be optimally utilized in order to guarantee an optimal OR efficiency.

OR information systems should – in order to support an optimal OR efficiency – be able to allocate (by scheduling ànd by managing) the optimal amount of OR time for every surgeon in order to minimize the sum of the costs of the unused OR time and to minimize the costs of elective cases being performed outside their normal allocated OR times. Optimal OR efficiency should by guided by an OR information system enabling centralized scheduling, daily management of OR activity and posthoc evaluation of OR activity by analysing all registered data in balanced scorecards [4,5].

In the present paper, we describe how the introduction of such an OR information management system influenced the efficiency of our daily OR activity.

1. Methodology

1.1. General Methodology

Since January 2001 we introduced a dynamic informatisation tool (Operating Room Management module) as a guide to everyday's OR management in 16 operating theatres at 3 different sites (Ziekenhuis Oost-Limburg with campus St Jan in Genk, campus André Dumont in Waterschei and campus St Barbara in Lanaken). ORM-m is part of the Yuse Matrix Box, which is an integrated cross-department software package for hospital's primary care processes. The Operating Room Management module is one of their departmental modules that, next to its primary objectives of providing a guide to OR management, also provides access to all underlying functionalities (electronic orders, planning and appointments, medical records and medical archive). The key component of the Operating Room Management module is an airport-like screen, displaying all scheduled OR activity pro OR theatre, linked in real-time activity with all OR theatres, where predefined tracking events (especially start (in) and end (out) of operation) are captured. As already described, we implemented this OR information system, as part of this central hospital information system, with interactive link to all administrative, all medical and all nursing data available in the hospital.

In order to realize the dynamic features, necessary for optimal OR efficiency, the OR information system was build around 3 major parts, consisting of centralized electronic scheduling of all OR procedures, daily management of all OR activity and balanced scorecards.

1.2. Centralized Electronic Scheduling of OR Procedures by OR-Planner

First, the ORM-m contains an interactive centralized electronic scheduling of OR procedures (OR-Planner), by offering a general OR agenda assigning allocated block times for all surgical groups [6-10]. From their surgical booking offices (as well in- as out-doors the hospital) surgeons enter all necessary information (for patient ànd procedure) concerning the actual scheduling of an OR procedure into the OR-Planner. In the same time, this scheduling evenso enables to reserve the patient's bed (in-hospital facility – short- or long-stay- or day clinic facility). All information provided by the surgical scheduling is readily available for the OR management staff and is displayed on a dynamic "airport"-screen, as part of the OR information system.

1.3. Airport-Screen as Management Tool to Daily OR Management

Secondly, during daily OR-activity, the ORM-m guides, by the means of a visual display screen, daily OR management by real-time registration of all OR "times" in all OR theatres [11,12]. This implicates an automatic registration of patients entering the operating room (in OR) and patients leaving the operating room (out OR). These "in-out" registrations provide the central OR-activity display (airport)-screen with updated information on actual activity. The difference in time between out OR and in OR results in the total real OR time registered for every OR procedure. The knowledge of the real total OR time registered for each OR procedure is an essential element in determining optimum OR utilization [11].

Next to time registration, there is also an electronic registration of all OR materials and medications, used during the OR procedure. This automatic registration is linked to the information system supporting the activity of the pharmacy department. At time of scheduling, all necessary OR medications and materials are predefined, referring to the specific OR profile (=surgeon + specific OR code). These predefined defaults are prepared at time of scheduling and are automatically transmitted to the pharmacy department. At the end of the operative procedure, these defaults are confirmed or are modified, and then final confirmation and facturation by the pharmacy department can be immediately performed [13].

A central displayed airport-screen offers an immediate overview of current, passed and to-be-performed OR-activity. This central screen is connected to the automatic time registration performed in all OR theatres (at 3 different sites) and offers an immediate up-dated view of ongoing OR activity. This dynamic screen offers moreover the possibility to a rapid scheduling (by the OR management staff) of urgent (or semi-urgent) procedures, and to a user-friendly re-scheduling of procedures from the central airport-screen, without the necessity to enter into the respective surgical booking modules (OR-planner).

The airport-screen also displays all necessary information on hospital admission (specific surgical ward), pre-operative anesthesia-screening, post-operative ICU admission etc.... by simple visual effects (icons) displayed on the screen. It also provides an immediate link to all medical results, protocols and documents of the respective patients (e.g. access to digital x-ray data readily availably to the surgeon in the operating theatre).

This dynamic overview of OR activity is available as a central information system through all hospital departments that have any connection to OR activity, e.g. surgical wards, postanesthesia care unit, intensive care units, day clinics, pharmacy department, sterilization department.....[14]

1.4. Analysis of all Registered Data in Balanced Scorecards

Thirdly, at the end of a day of OR activity, all registered data on OR utilization become available. These raw data are analyzed by pre-defined queries to obtain immediate balanced scorecards. In the same time, any significant change compared to previously obtained results, is automatically analyzed, in order to anticipate or to immediate intervene in case of any trend change. These balanced scorecards are generally divided into operational and quality balanced scorecards. The operational scorecards include information on the number of surgical interventions / OR code / surgeon; the average case duration / OR code / surgeon; the utilization ratio / surgeon / surgical block time; the scheduled versus the actual case duration / OR code /surgeon; the excess-time / surgeon / surgical discipline; the underutilized time / surgeon / surgical discipline. The quality balanced scorecards offer as well quality insights for patient's well-being as quality insights into the surgical procedures themselves.

The immediate availability of readily interpretable balanced scorecards offers an unique opportunity to immediate fine-tuning of OR management, in view of any changes influencing the overall OR activity and efficiency [15].

Before the introduction of ORM-m, all scheduling of OR activity was assembled and guided by the OR head nurse, who obtained all necessary information from the surgeon or on paper (typed or hand-written) or by telephone. All obtained information was then written down in the central "OR-book". During daily OR-activity, all time notifications, all materials and medication were registered on papers (written down by the OR nurses). Afterwards, all registered data were entered into excell-files by OR-administrative personal.

After the introduction of our current ORM-m system in our hospital, we wanted to illustrate its influence on the overall OR efficiency. For the purpose of this paper, we analyzed all OR data registered for just one surgical discipline (abdominal surgery) before and after the introduction of the information system. Statistical analysis was performed using the Mann-Whitney U-test.

2. Results

For this paper, we compared all data of OR activity for elective (excluding all urgent and semi-urgent cases) abdominal surgery for the first half of 2000 to the first half of 2001 (just after the introduction of the ORM-m). Urgent and semi-urgent cases were excluded from this analysis as these cases are not scheduled by the surgeons themselves but by the OR management staff at request of the surgeon. In our instution, urgent cases are defined as procedures that have to be performed within 6 hours from acknowledgement, whereas semi-urgent cases can wait for as long as 24 hours, but anyhow they are not scheduled by the surgeons themselves as the (electronic) OR-planner is closed at 36 hours before surgery.

From January to June 2000, 764 elective cases were performed, whereas 815 elective cases were performed from January to June 2001. For both periods, the total OR block time allocated to abdominal surgery for this 6 months period was the same, namely 805 hrs.

For 2000, the total duration of OR activity registered for elective abdominal surgery was 1044h50min (this means 239h50min over-time, or more than the allocated 895 hours), whereas for 2001 we registered a total of 1127h35min (implicating 322h35min over-time).

For 2000, we recorded 147h20min excess-time (= exceeding the normal time limits of OR activity – from 8.00 am until 16.30 pm- and inducing extra costs) and 46h45min unused OR time. For 2001, we recorded 123h04min excess-time and 35h21min unused time.

This means that for 2001, reviewing all data concerning elective abdominal surgery, we observed an non-significant increase in the total number of cases performed (from 764 to 815 or +6.6%), with significant less excess-time (123h04min vs 147h20min or –16.3%), partly explained by a significant reduction in unused OR time (35h21min for 2001 compared to 46h45min for 2000 or – 23%).

After further analysis of the balances scorecards, the significant reduction in unused OR time can partly be explained by a significant reduction in turnover time (defined as the time lap between previous patient out of OR and next patient in OR). Mean turnover time registered (on paper) for 2000 was 12.3 min, whereas for 2001 we registered (electronically) a mean turnover time of 7.8 min. The observed decrease in turnover time could partly be caused by a methodological change in registration mode (electronic registration vs hand-written registration).

	2000	2001
Nr operative procedures	764	815
Total hours available	805h	805h
Total duration of all procedures	1044h50min	1127h35min*
Total excess-time	147h20min	123h04min*
Total unused-time	46h45min	35h21min*

However next to these methodological changes, we also observed a significant reduction in arrival time from ward to OR. For 2000, we registered mean arrival times from ward to OR of 21.32 min, whereas for 2001, this time significantly decreased to 14.15 min.

3. Discussion

The observed improvement in OR efficiency should be explained by many factors. Most importantly, it should be interpreted as well in view of the introduction of an information system allowing centralized scheduling of OR procedures as in view of the introduction of an information system displaying a real-time overview on general OR activity over all theatres, throughout the whole hospital, enabling optimal utilization of all disposable OR time ànd registration of all relevant data, ultimately available for analysis by balanced scorecards. Information systems introduced for cost- and quality-management of daily OR-activity should support all items of OR-activity from scheduling to management (4). Information systems only partly supporting OR-activity, such as anesthesia information management systems, can only partly alleviate and guide daily OR management [5,16,17].

3.1. How to Interprete the Role of Centralized Electronic Scheduling?

For already a long time, literature revealed that centralized OR scheduling, enabling to book surgical procedures as well as to reserve hospital beds, was more performant than decentralized scheduling of OR procedures [21-23]. All authors reported a rise in utilization of OR rooms when centralized OR scheduling was applied compared to a decentralized system of OR scheduling. So for sure, the "central and electronic booking opportunity" of our OR information system could have taken a great part in the observed improvement of OR efficiency.

The electronic OR-planner, opening all allocated block time to direct scheduling from the surgical booking offices, resulted for sure in a more accurate (as well concerning patient- as procedure-identification) and in a more complete information transmission to the OR management staff compared to the former way of transmission before 2001.

The fact that the scheduling of an OR procedure in the OR-planner also includes the use of predefined defaults, referring to the specific OR profile, off all necessary OR materials and medication and the transmission of these data to the pharmacy department, supports a just in time inventory control of all necessary material and medication [13]. This improvement in material- and medication-management might also have contributed to the observed improvement in OR efficiency (e.g. no long waiting times anymore during operation in case of inavailibility of some specific OR material).

3.2. How to Interprete the Role of an "Overall" Available Screen, Displaying Real-Time OR Activity?

The introduction of an airport-like screen, containing all scheduled information, and directed by real-time registration from all OR theatres, changed our daily OR management extensively, compared to the previous situation with just a hand-written OR book as daily guide. Moreover, the visual display of all registered events, comprehensible for every participant, enabled pro-active and accurate management, clearly reducing unused OR-time.

The immediate access (in all OR theatres) to all medical data (results, protocols…) offers the best condition for pre-operative, pre-anesthesia preparation. The fact that there were no missing results anymore might also have improved total OR efficiency.

The availability of the ORM-m airport-like screen throughout the whole hospital, offering a way of direct communication between all participants in OR activity, also plays a major role in the observed results [14]. The reduction in arrival time from ward to OR can mainly be attributed to this "open-house" strategy, thanks to the hospital wide availability of the OR-screen. Nurses on the surgical wards have immediate access to daily ongoing OR-activity and anticipate to prepare their patients for surgical intervention, as they do not longer wait for the final call from the OR. This anticipation is one of the main factors that induced a reduction in arrival time from ward to OR, thereby reducing turnover time and finally reducing unused OR time [18-20].

3.3. How to Interprete the Final Results from Balanced Scorecards?

All data registered by OR-Planner and ORM-m, concerning as well the scheduling information as concerning the daily OR activity-information, are used for analysis by balanced scorecards. Predefined queries can be obtained [15] and statistical analysis of different elements of OR utilization can be performed. Use of these balanced scorecards for the analysis of the cases performed for elective abdominal surgery comparing the first half of 2000 to the first half of 2001, revealed a (non-significant) increase in number of procedures performed. This increase did however not incur at the expense of an increase in OR costs, thanks to a better use of available OR-time, with less excess-time and less unused OR-time.

4. Conclusions

Information systems designed to guide OR management should support all aspects of OR activity. Informatisation of OR management starts with centralized electronic scheduling, enables the management of daily OR-activity by a visual display of all real-time ongoing OR activity and results in the analysis of all registered data by predefined queries for balanced scorecards. In this paper, we illustrated how the introduction of ORM-m supported electronic central scheduling of all our OR procedures and guided our daily OR management. As a final result, from the balanced scorecards, we observed an overall improved OR efficiency, with more procedures performed at less expenses.

References

[1] Macario A, Vitez TS, Dunn B, McDonald T. Where are the costs in perioperative care? Analysis of hospital costs and charges for inpatient surgical care. Anesthesiology 1995;83:1138-1144.

[2] Roberts RR, Frutos PW, Ciavarella GG, Gussow LM, Mensah EK, Kampe LM, Straus HE, Joseph G, Rydman RJ. Distribution of variable vs fixed costs of hospital care. JAMA 1999;281:644-649.

[3] Abouleish AE, Dexter F, Whitten CW, Zavaleta JR, Prough DS. Quantifying net staffing costs due to longer-than-average surgical case durations. Anesthesiology 2004;100:403-412.

[4] Warnock-Matheron AG, Hannah KJ. Comparative analysis of computer-based operating room information systems : an evaluation research study. Computers in Nursing. 1988;6:147-156.

[5] Junger A, Benson M, Quinzio L, Michel A, Sciuk G, Brammen D, Marquardt K, Hempelmann G. An Anesthesia Information Management System as a tool for controlling resource management of operating rooms. Methods of Information in Medicine 2002;41:81-85.

[6] Blake JT, Dexter F, Donald J. Operating room managers'use of integer programming for assigning allocated block time to surgical groups : a case study. Anesthesia & Analgesia 2002;94:143-148.

[7] Dexter F, Macario A. Applications of information systems to operating room scheduling. Anesthesiolology 1996;85:1232-1234.

[8] Ozkarahan I. Allocation of surgical procedures to operating rooms. Journal of Medical Systems. 1995;19:333-352.

[9] Strum DP, Vargas LG, May JH, Bashein G. Surgical suite utilization and capacity planning : a minimal cost analysis model. Journal of Medical Systems 1997;21:309-322.
[10] Kuo PC, Schroeder RA, Mahaffey S, Bollinger RR. Optimization of operating room allocation using linear programming techniques. Journal of the American College of Surgeons 2003;197:889-895.
[11] Tyler DC, Pasquariello CA, Chen CH. Determining optimum operating room utilization. Anesthesia&Analgesia 2003;96:1114-1121.
[12] Weinbroum AA. Efficiency of the operating room suite. The American Journal of Surgery 2003;185:244-250.
[13] Epstein RH, Dexter F. Economic analysis of linking operating room scheduling and hospital materal management information systems for just in time inventory control. Anesthesia&Analgesia 2000;91:337-343.
[14] Moss J, Xia Y. Improving operating room coordination : communication pattern assessment. The Journal of Nursing Administration 2004;34:93-100.
[15] Dexter F, Epstein RH, Marsh HM. Statistical analysis of weekday operating room anesthesia group staffing independently managed surgical suites. Anesthesia & Analgesia 2001;92:1493-1498.
[16] Dexter F, Macario A, Traub RD, Hopwood M, Lubarsky DA. An operating room scheduling strategy to maximize the use of operating room block time – Computer simulation of patient scheduling and survey of patients' preferences for surgical waiting times. Anesthesia&Analgesia 1999;89:7-20.
[17] Dexter F, Macario A, Lubarsky DA. Impact on revenue of increasing patient volume at surgical suite with relatively high operating room utilization. Anesthesia&Analgesia 2001;92:1215-1221.
[18] Champault A, Arsena V, Barrat C, Bayeh P, Champault G. Can the time between interventions be reduced in the operating theatre ? AnnChir 2003;128:599-602.
[19] Dexter F, Abouleish AE, Epstein RH, Whitten CW, Lubarsky DA. Use of operating room information system data predicts the impact of reducing turnover times on staffing costs. Anesthesia&Analgesia 2003;97:1119-1126.
[20] Adams R, Warner P, Hubbard B, Goulding T. Decreasing turnaround time between general surgery cases. Journal of Nursing Administration 2004;34:140-148.
[21] Lowry JC, Martin JB. Evaluation of an advance surgical scheduling system. Journal of Medical Systems 1989;13:11-23.
[22] McQuarrie DG. Limits of efficient operating room scheduling. Lessons learned from computer-use models. Archives of Surgery 1981;116:1065-1071.
[23] Przasnyski ZH. Operating room scheduling : a literature review. AORN Journal 1986;44:67-79.

Contact Address:

Cathy S.I. De Deyne, MD PhD
Dept of Anesthesia and Critical Care Medicine
Ziekenhuis Oost-Limburg
Schiepse Bos 6
3600 Genk – Belgium

"The Declaration of Innsbruck": Some Reflections

Jan L. TALMON[a] and Elske AMMENWERTH[b]
[a]*Department of Medical Informatics, Maastricht University, Maastricht*
[b]*Research Group Assessment of Health Information Systems, University for Health Sciences, Medical Informatics and Technology (UMIT), Austria*

Abstract. In 2003 a workshop was held in Innsbruck, Austria, on the topic of evaluation of ICT applications in Health Care. A result of that workshop was the "Declaration of Innsbruck". In the current paper we will further elaborate on this declaration and discuss some of the activities that are currently undertaken as supportive measures to enable the realization of the vision expressed in the declaration.

Keywords. Evaluation, ICT, Declaration of Innsbruck, GEP-HI, STARE-HI, EP-HI

Introduction

Evaluation of health ICT applications is a topic of concern. Decision makers are seeking information that will support ICT investment decisions. Policy makers are looking for evidence whether the implemented systems produce the anticipated results. A recent report of the Institute for Public Policy Research (IPPR) in England has identified a number of problems in relation of the British National Programme for IT in the NHS [1]. In this report several reasons for the lack of evidence are listed:

- Maybe there are real problems with how ICT is used.
- Maybe we are not looking for the evidence properly.

The last point was further elucidated by statements like: too little time and too little resources were allocated to evaluation; the rationale for the evaluation was unclear; no sufficient data are present to enable evaluation of ICT; inadequate methods were used.

The interest in evaluation of ICT dates back till the early nineties. In Europe several projects have been addressing the issue. Without being complete, useful results have been presented by e.g. the ATIM project [2] and IMIA's Working Groups 13&15 working conference in Helsinki [3]. In 2003 a group of experts on evaluation with various backgrounds convened in Innsbruck, Austria, to further elaborate on the issue. One of the results of the conference was the Declaration of Innsbruck, which has been published in 2004 [4]. In the current paper, we will further elaborate on the declaration, taking into account several discussions with researchers from all over the world at the MEDINFO 2004 conference in San Francisco.

1. The Declaration of Innsbruck

1.1. The Preamble

The declaration starts with a preamble that defines why evaluation is a necessary activity.

"Health Information Systems are intended to improve the functioning of health professionals and organisations in managing health and delivering healthcare. Given the significance of this type of intervention, and the intended beneficial effect on patients and professionals, it is morally imperative to ensure that the optimum results are achieved, and any unanticipated outcomes identified. The necessary process is ***evaluation****, and this should be considered an essential adjunct to design and implementation of information systems."*

This statement is in line with the observations in the IPPR report. Also at MEDINFO 2004 it has been stressed that implementing a Health Information System without a proper evaluation is bad practice.

As to further elaborate on this issue, the declaration consists of three parts: Definitions, Observations and Recommendations.

1.2. The Definitions

The definition part has been included to make clear that a health information system is more that a pure technological system.

§I. A ***system*** *is a set of components (e.g., actors and artifacts), [...], which as a whole is needed to accomplish an objective. A health information system (HIS) comprises actors [...] and artifacts [...] that together process health-related information in a health care organization. It operates in an organizational environment made up of people (e.g. system developers, politicians, managers, patients) and procedures, which influence its development and operation.*

From this definition it is clear that a too narrow conception of a HIS may lead to a technocratic approach that will not take into account the actors that need to work with the technology nor the others that are affected by the use of the technology.

The second definition deals with evaluation:

§II. ***Evaluation*** *is the act of measuring or exploring properties of a health information system (in planning, in development, in implementation, or in operation), the result of which informs a decision to be made concerning that system in a specific context. Evaluation of health information systems has to deal with the actors, the artefacts, and their interaction to best support the decisions to be made.*

The most important element in this definition is that evaluation is done with a purpose. Without such a purpose evaluation has no value. It further makes explicit that all components of the HIS have to be taken into account. It is commonly accepted that an evaluation could address one or more of the following aspects: technical, clinical, organisational, economic, psychological/sociological, ethical, and legal.

1.3. The Observations

(i) Evaluation generates information to improve knowledge and to generate insight.
Although this observation may seem self-evident, publications on evaluation studies not always make explicit what knowledge or insight has been gained from the study. In particu-

lar earlier studies on decision support systems and classification algorithms have often only reported on their accuracy. The authors seldom refer to what has been learned.

(ii) Evaluation supports reflective practice.
This is a very important observation in our view. It expresses a professional attitude that each medical informatician should embrace. Each and every professional should reflect on his or her activities. Evaluation helps to assess to what degree one adheres e.g. to ethical engineering principles. It is important to notice that doing evaluations also furthers the development of evidence-based medical informatics.

(iii) Evaluation is a challenging endeavour.
The fact that validated evaluation frameworks and evaluation methodologies are largely lacking is an indication that evaluation isn't an easy task. Since many actors and artifacts may be involved and since there are many dimensions to consider in an evaluation, clear guidelines on how to set-up and execute an evaluation study are difficult to develop. Those that are available approach the topic from a high level. They provide general guidance, but when it comes to what precisely to measure and how these guidelines fall short. A factor that further complicates the issue is that the various methods and techniques that could be applied do not necessarily come from the field of medicine or computer science. Some techniques have their roots in sociology, psychology, business science etc. Research paradigms from the health sciences should be considered as well.

(iv) Evaluation is not free.
Evaluation is expensive. It is not something to "just do at the end of the project to see whether it is successful". Evaluation has to be planned carefully and resources have to be allocated. On the other hand, the results of the evaluation do have a value as well. Not necessarily in monetary terms. Evaluations provide knowledge and insight about the complex processes that takes place in health care. We may become better prepared when new applications are being conceived, developed and implemented. Evaluation results that inform decision makers in the proper way could save a significant amount of money when they reduce the chance of making improper decisions. This observation entails that the earlier evaluation can inform decision makers, the best chance exist that the available resources are spend as good as possible.

1.4. The Recommendations

Some of the recommendations follow directly from the observations made above. Others are based on experiences of the various participants at the Innsbruck workshop.

1. *Evaluation should be seen as an ethical imperative.*

This recommendation follows directly from observation (ii). As argued above ethics are relevant. In the code of ethics adopted by IMIA, there are statements about evaluation [5]:

> *[Health Information Professionals] ... have a duty to ensure, to the best of their ability, that appropriate structures are in place to evaluate the technical, legal and ethical acceptability of the data-collection, storage, retrieval, processing, accessing, communication, and utilization of data in the settings in which they carry out their work or with which they are affiliated.*

Although this statement is written in the context of electronic records, it is equally applicable for any artefact that manipulates patient data, including decision support systems. This statement has been written to protect the patient, but it is also relevant to protect the user of the system, i.e. the health care professional. Evaluations should demonstrate that the HIS environment is safe, efficient and effective to work with.

2. *Evaluation should be sufficiently funded.*

Appropriate resources should be made available for evaluation. It should be part of the budget. There should be no pressure to reallocate evaluation funds to development. It is attractive to spend some more money to improve the artefacts, but when it cannot be proven that they are effective due to the limited resources left, the whole endeavour has to be considered as a failure. It will erode trust and in the end fund givers may become reluctant to invest in ICT in health care due to the lack of evidence of impact.

3. *Evaluators should be free from pressure.*

Some stakeholders may have an interest in a certain outcome of an evaluation study. The evaluator should, however, be guarded from any pressure with respect to the conclusions of a study. The evaluator should perform a study based on his or her professional expertise. During the design of the study, the evaluator may have to negotiate with the study commissioner on the depth and breadth of a study. The evaluator should honestly discuss the value of the study in relation with the funds available. As soon as the evaluation plan has been agreed, the evaluator should be free from any pressure to present his findings and to bend his conclusions in any specific direction.

4. *Evaluation studies should be grounded on scientific theory and rigorous approaches.*

Evaluation should be evidence based. The best available methods and techniques should be used and applied in any given situation. What method to choose will of course also depend on the actual problem at hand. Doing evaluations based only on rigorous scientific theory will enhance the credibility of the evaluations. Such an approach will contribute to building an evidence base for Medical Informatics as a profession.

5. *Evaluation methods should be selected with an open mind.*

Every evaluator has been educated with a particular research paradigm. Since evaluation is multi-facetted the evaluator should in the selection of methods not be restricted to that paradigm. Evaluators should be open to methods and approaches from other disciplines and adopt those that are appropriate for the task at hand. This entails that evaluators should have a broad knowledge of various disciplines. When detailed knowledge is needed, the evaluator should involve professionals with the background needed.

6. *Reports on methodological and methodical studies[1] should be encouraged.*

There is a need to expand the methodological arsenal for evaluation. The validity of methods and approaches need to be established. Also the application range and limitations need to be documented as to support evaluators in the choice of the appropriate approach in a given situation. Without a proper evidence base and scientific grounding of the various methods it is difficult for the evaluator to act professionally. Personal preferences would then reign the field. Specifically the integration of various (qualitative and quantitative) methods in a multi-method framework is a challenging task.

7. *Guidelines for good evaluation practice should be made available.*

Guidelines can assist evaluators in selecting and applying the best methods according to existing evidence. Comprehensive guidelines for good evaluation practice hardly exist. Only rather general approaches have suggested[6-8]. Further work in this area is needed. Guidelines should state the strength of the evidence for the recommendations given.

8. *Terms, concepts and guidelines for reporting on results of ICT assessment studies should be developed.*

Current literature on evaluation studies varies largely in quality. Sufficient information is seldom present to assess the value of a study. Methodological issues are hardly dealt with.

This reduces the value and credibility of the studies. To improve the evidence base of Medical Informatics more rigorous reporting of assessment studies are needed. We should also avoid using concepts and terms that are poorly defined. Only when we are able to define and apply the proper language and structure of evaluation studies reports we will build up evidence that is open to broad use, including meta-analysis.

9. Evaluation should be promoted by centres of excellence.

Good evaluation practice is not only relevant for the scientific development of Medical Informatics. It is also relevant for the Health Care industry. Promotion of good evaluation practice is therefore a useful endeavour. Centres of excellence could play a role in this. To avoid conflicts of interest such centres should operate on a not-for-profit basis and be independent of providers of specific ICT for health care. Only then they can provide independent consultancy on evaluation.

10. Evaluation networks should be established.

(Inter-)national collaboration in evaluation is needed. Developing guidelines and building an evidence base are sincere efforts that require broad input. Social and cultural differences should be made explicit. A network of interested parties will provide a community in which evaluation research can foster. Since the multi-disciplinary nature of evaluation such networks should cover professionals with different backgrounds as to provide the broad spectrum of disciplines that is needed to further the field.

11. An open access repository about evaluation studies should be established.

Experiences of others could inform decision makers about potential pitfalls and dead alleys that should be avoided. A good evidence base on which strategies work and which not is invaluable. Such an evidence base would assist evaluators to design studies that avoid pitfalls that may lead to failed assessment. It could also be of value as a repository of success and failure criteria for implementation of ICT in health care.

12. Appreciation of methods of evaluation should be part of health informatics curricula.

Each medical informatican should have at least a basic knowledge of methodologies and methods necessary to accomplish evaluation of HIS. However to be a professional evaluator requires further study and a broad experience.

2. Current Activities

The EFMI working group on Evaluation together with the IMIA working group on Technology Assessment and Quality Improvement have taken the lead in addressing several issues listed above. There is a major interest around the world in these endeavours. The Evaluation working group of AMIA is recently established and is joining in. Three activities are worth mentioning in this context.

2.1. GEP-HI

GEP-HI aims at the development of guidelines for good evaluation practice in health informatics. Recent discussions have lead to the insight that one comprehensive guideline is next to impossible to develop. GEP-HI is likely to develop a series of guidelines that address either global approaches to assessment or more detailed and focussed aspects, e.g. with respect to economic evaluations.

2.2. STARE-HI

The objective of STARE-HI is to develop standards for the reporting of evaluation studies in Health Informatics. This activity is inspired by the work on the CONSORT [9] and STARD [10] statements as developed for reporting of medical research. Plans are to develop a brief statement on how evaluation studies should be reported and an accompanying document in which evidence is provided why the various recommendations are made.

2.3. EP-HI

One means to achieve the goal of open access to evaluation studies is to develop an evaluation portal. The objective of such a portal is not only to provide access to study results. It aims at being a "one-stop shopping" area for all kind of issues related to evaluation. Two developments take currently place. Firstly a website is being developed. A proof of concept is available at http://toolbox.unimaas.nl/. Secondly, activities are undertaken to secure the financial basis of such a site.

Currently the site points to various guidelines (ATIM book, VATAM, PROBE). A rather extensive glossary of terms is present. A link has been setup to a database with over 1000 references to evaluation studies, maintained at UMIT, Austria. An endeavour is made to get the comprehensive description of a set of over 30 evaluation methods translated into English. This will be the core of the "methods" section of EP-HI. We are also working on collecting questionnaires that are of relevance for the evaluation of ICT in health care.

3. Summary

We presented the main statements of the declaration of Innsbruck dealing with evaluation issues in Health Informatics. We elaborated the reasons for the various observations and recommendations. We presented current developments at a European level to realize some of the recommendations of the declaration. During MEDINFO 2004 it was decided by the AMIA working group to critically assess the declaration and to make suggestions for improvement. The final goal is to have the declaration broadly adopted.

Endnote

[1] 'Methodology' means the 'knowledge (logos) of methods', i.e. how to deal with methods, while 'methodical' means that methods are stringently applied.

References

[1] J. Bend (2004): Public Value and e-Health, Institute for Public Policy Research. http://www.ippr.org/research/files/team34/project143/Bend_PublicValueandeHealth_ippr.pdf, last visited: 11 September 2004.

[2] E.M.S.J. van Gennip, J.L. Talmon, editors (1995): Assessment and Evaluation of Information Technologies in Medicine. *Studies in Health Technology and Informatics. Amsterdam: IOS Press.*

[3] J.L. Talmon, N. Lorenzi, E.M.S.J. van Gennip, P. Nykänen (1999): Organisational issues and technology assessment in health informatics - Editorial. *Int J Med Inform; 56 1-2.*

[4] E. Ammenwerth, J. Brender, P. Nykänen, H.-U. Prokosch, M. Rigby, J. Talmon: (2004) Visions and strategies to improve evaluation of health information systems: Reflections and lessons based on the HIS-EVAL workshop in Innsbruck. *Int J Med Inform; 73, 479-491.*

[5] IMIA Code of Ethics for Health Information Professionals. http://www.imia.org/English_code_of_ethics.html, last visited 11 September 2004.

[6] J.L. Talmon, J. Enning, G. Castaneda, F. Eurlings, D. Hoyer, P. Nykänen, F. Sanz, C. Thayer, M. Vissers (1999): The VATAM guidelines. *Int J Med Inform 1999; 107-115.*
[7] Probe toolkit, http://www.it-p.net/probe/ Last visited 14 september 2004.
[8] A.P. Stoop, M. Berg (2004): Integrating quantitative and qualitative methods in patient care information system evaluation: Guidance for the organizational decision maker. *Meth Inf Med, 42, 458-462.*
[9] M.K. Campbell, D.R. Elbourne, D.G. Altman for the CONSORT Group (2004): CONSORT statement: extension to cluster randomised trials. *BMJ 328, 702-708.*
[10] P.M. Bossuyt; J.B. Reitsma; D.E. Bruns; C.A. Gatsonis; P.P. Glasziou; L.M. Irwig; J.G. Lijmer; D. Moher; D. Rennie; and H.C.W. de Vet, for the STARD Group (2003): Towards Complete and Accurate Reporting of Studies of Diagnostic Accuracy: The STARD Initiative. *Ann Int Med, 138, 40-44.*

Contact address

J.L. Talmon
Dept. of Medical Informatics
Maastricht University
PO box 616
6200MD Maastricht
The Netherlands
Tel: +31 43 3882243
Email: Talmon@mi.unimaas.nl

Testing the ISO Nursing Reference Terminology Model for Mapping

William GOOSSEN
Acquest Research and Development,
Dorpsstraat 50 2396 HC Koudekerk aan den Rijn, the Netherlands

Abstract. Purpose: The ISO IS 18104 is intended for helping the nursing profession to integrate their terminologies into computer systems and into larger health care reference terminologies. One purpose of the standard is to map between different terminologies.

Method: This mapping was tested, using three terminologies that are relevant for nursing in the Netherlands. Concepts and terms where selected, and their equivalence was determined by experts, and next these were dissected.

Results: The dissection revealed that several concepts can easily be interchanged among the three example terminologies, while others cannot, or only for specific purposes.

Conclusions: The ISO IS 18104 fulfills this purpose very well and can be considered the gold standard for mapping of nursing terminologies.

Keywords. Nursing terminology, reference model, classification, standardization, nursing minimum data set, nursing information management

Introduction

One outcome of international collaboration of nursing professionals in the area of terminology, health information standards and nursing informatics is the current ISO standard IS 18104 [1]. This is based on earlier European standardization work [2, 3]. The IS 18104 'a reference terminology model for nursing' was approved in 2003 and its main purpose is to establish a nursing reference terminology model consistent with the goals and objectives of other specific health terminology models in order to provide a more unified reference health model. This International Standard includes the development of reference terminology models for nursing diagnoses and nursing actions and relevant terminology and definitions for its implementation.

The potential uses for this reference terminology model are to:

- support the intensional definition of nursing diagnosis and nursing action concepts,
- facilitate the representation of nursing diagnosis and action concepts and their relationships for computer processing,
- provide a framework for generating compositional expressions from atomic concepts within a reference terminology,
- facilitate the construction of nursing terminologies which makes mapping easier,
- facilitate the mapping among nursing diagnosis and nursing action concepts from various terminologies,
- enable the systematic evaluation of terminologies and associated terminology models, and

- provide a language to describe the structure of nursing diagnosis and nursing action concepts to enable integration with other reference terminology models, and with information models [1].

The model helps for instance in mapping nursing terminologies into larger health and medical terminologies [4, 5]. The standard has been tested for nursing interventions and for nursing diagnoses [4, 5, 6]. Moss et al [6] checked the quality of nursing interventions in documentation and Bakken et al [4] used the ISO model for inclusion of nursing concepts into SNOMED CT, and Hwang et al to integrate nursing diagnostic concepts into a medical dictionary [5].

This paper reports the test of the ISO standard IS 18104 for its usefulness for supporting mapping between two health classifications and the items of the Dutch nursing minimum data set (NMDSN). In this test, both the application of terminologies for clinical use, and for aggregate purposes is taken into account. The NMDSN is intended to aggregate information from clinical nursing documentation that is based on health classifications [7, 8]. If the mapping is adequate, this helps in aggregating nursing information from individual patient records for aggregate purposes. If the concepts are sufficiently matching, they also can be interchanged in nursing practice, for instance, in electronic messages.

1. Method

This ISO IS 18104 represents the semantic definitions of nursing concepts, relationships between these concepts and the attributes of their characteristics. Figure 1 contains the ISO model for nursing diagnoses. A nursing diagnosis must have a focus, which is an area of attention, for example 'breathing pattern', 'pain', 'activities of daily living', or 'social skills'. One optional attribute for focus is timing. Focus has a relationship with site (e.g., pain has site leg) and has a relationship with the subject of information, e.g. the individual, a group or other. The second mandatory part of a nursing diagnosis is the judgment of the nurse, for instance 'problematic' or 'limited', which is applied to the focus. In addition, the judgment can be enhanced with detail about degree of severity, actual or potential, or acute or chronic. Dimension is useful for further specification; it can be a perspective on the focus. For example if the focus is the patients' activity of daily living, dimension can be used to define the detail, such as clothing, toileting among others.

To test the IS 18104 for its mapping capabilities, the following procedure was carried out. Three sample terminological systems were selected. These are the Nursing Minimum Data Set the Netherlands (NMDSN) [7, 8], the International Classification for Nursing

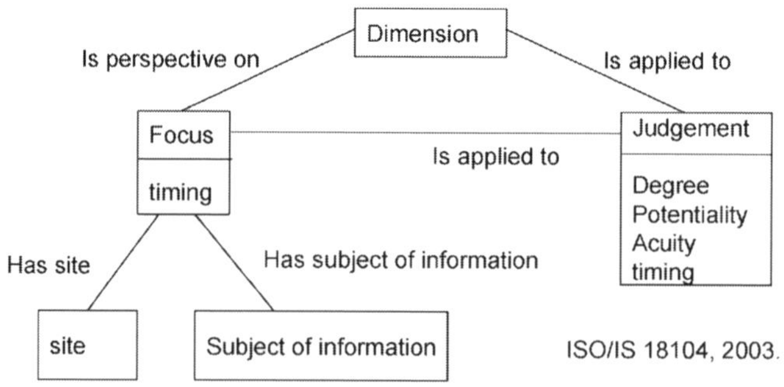

Figure 1. The ISO reference terminology model for nursing diagnoses [1].

Practice (ICNP® Beta 2) [9], and the International Classification of Functioning, Disability and Health (ICF) [10].

The NMDSN has been developed and tested to describe the diversity of patient populations and the variation of nursing practice, and to calculate nursing workload [7, 8]. NMDSN consists of patient demographics, setting items, nursing diagnosis, interventions and some results of nursing care.

The ICNP® is developed by the International Council of Nurses (ICN), with large financial support from the EU Telenurse project [9]. It consists of two multi-axial classifications. The first multi-axial part contains concepts to describe nursing phenomena. Nurses can use these concepts to document nursing diagnoses. The ICNP® consists of about 685 concepts for the focus of nursing care, and 334 concepts for nursing judgments. The other axes contain roughly 250 concepts that serve as qualifiers for frequency, duration, topology, anatomical location, likelihood and bearer. The basic structure of the ISO model is largely based on the ICNP®. Each ICNP® axis has a hierarchical structure in which the concepts are organised and coded. Due to the combinatorial possibilities, the ICNP® is often referred to as the nursing maximum data set. It allows describing many thousands of patient problems. The second part of ICNP® consists of about 1500 concepts to describe nursing actions. The ICNP® functions as a combinatorial terminology for nursing practice and provides a unifying framework into which local language and existing nursing terminologies and classifications can be cross-mapped [11].

The ICF is developed by the WHO and offers a structure and a classification of more than thousand concepts describing human functioning [10]. The concepts are classified, coded and defined according to three perspectives on human functioning. These are the functions and structures of the human body, activities of the human being, and the participation of humans in society. Thus, the ICF structure consists of the following components, which are each organised in a hierarchical tree: Functions, Structures, Activities, Participation, External factors, and Personal factors. Unlike the ICNP®, the ICF has only one qualifier which consists of a scale on which the seriousness of the concept can be expressed (from no problem, via moderate problem, to major problem etc.).

Mapping in this study means the following: a NMDSN concept is compared with both a similar or comparable concept from the ICNP® Beta 2 version and from the ICF. Next, it is checked whether the terms and definitions have the same meaning. For the correct mapping (also referred to as mediation by Hardiker [12]) of NMDSN concepts from ICF and ICNP® equivalent concepts, terms and definitions are selected. In several cases this might imply that arbitrary choices must be made for particular terms from ICF and ICNP® that represent the NMDSN concepts as close as possible.

The following procedure was applied for mapping, loosely based on structural validation work of nursing terminologies by Hardiker and Rector [13]:

1. The 39 nursing diagnoses concepts from the NMDSN where put in a table.
2. From the ICF and ICNP® Beta 2 equivalent terms where chosen by the researcher.
3. Five external experts – three English speaking and two Dutch – validated the researcher's choices for equivalent terms.
4. The selected concepts were dissected according to the ISO model for nursing diagnoses.

Specifically, al concepts where analyzed according to the relevant elements as depicted in the ISO model. When all or almost all elements are equivalent between the concepts for the NMDSN and the two classifications, the mapping is adequate. Potentially, the terms can be interchanged between all three terminologies, so including between ICF and ICNP®. When these elements are not equivalent, further work is necessary to clarify the concepts and the terms and definitions that describe them.

An important aspect here is to determine at which level the possible problems with the semantics occur. This can be a problem at the clinical level: the granularity required for appropriate description of problems for the individual patient does not allow mapping. Alternatively, it can be at aggregate level: the differences in concepts might render it impossible to compare items for statistical purposes. Not all attributes of the ISO model where relevant for all concepts; therefore, in most occasions a selection was made.

2. Results

The results include information on semantic equivalence, dissections of equivalent terms, and insight in the extent to which concepts from the three terminologies can be interchanged. Thus, thirty-nine diagnostic concepts in the NMDSN are analyzed via the ISO standard.

2.1. Equivalence

Researcher and experts selected independently of each other and for each of the 39 diagnostic concepts in the NMDSN the equivalent term and definition from ICF and ICNP®. Decisions for equivalence are mainly based on focus, and sometimes on judgment. There are two concepts from the NMDSN that could not be matched at all: uncertainty about the future and insight in ones health situation. Further, some NMDSN items are not present in the ICF and not in the ICNP®. These are complications of investigations or treatment and accidents. These obviously have not been dissected. Examples of equivalent terms for focus are presented in Table 1.

2.2. Dissection of NMDSN Items

For those items about which the experts agree sufficiently, a dissection has been carried out based on the model for nursing diagnoses from the ISO standard. Example results are listed in Tables 2 & 3. An important finding is that the NMDSN concepts that concern problems of both the individual patient and the family or next of kin, cannot be compared with the ICF classification, because the ICF can only have the individual as subject of information. The ICNP® Beta 2 is equipped to express nursing diagnoses for groups because of an axis in which the bearer is described [9]. Upon choice, the kind of bearer can be used; individ-

Table 1. Examples for equivalent terms from NMDSN, ICNP® Beta 2 and ICF.

NMDSN item for focus:	ICF equivalent for focus:	ICNP® equivalent for focus:
3 Patient or family have fear	**b 1522 Range of emotion** Mental functions that produce the spectrum of experience of arousal of affect or feelings such as love, hate, anxiousness, sorrow, joy, fear and anger.	**1A.1.1.2.1.1.5.8 Fear** is a type of Emotion with the specific characteristics: Feelings of threat, danger or distress with known cause accompanied by alertness, concentration on the source of fear, wide-eyed aggressive attack mode of behaviour or withdrawal from source of fear.
8 Lack of motivation to co-operate in treatment and care	**b 1301 Motivation** Mental functions that produce the incentive to act; the conscious or unconscious driving force for action.	**1A.1.1.2.1 Reason for Action** is a type of Nursing Phenomenon of the Person with the specific characteristics: Motivation providing understanding and explanation for behaviour of the person.

Table 2. Dissection of the NMDSN concept 'patient or family have fear'.

NMDSN item	**ICF concept**	**ICNP® concepts**
Dissection:	**Dissection:**	**Dissection:**
has focus fear	has focus range of emotion (as part of emotional functions)	has focus fear
has judgment fear (meaning present)	has judgment impairment	has judgment demonstrates fear or fear yes, or decrease / increase of fear.
has subject of information patient and/or family	has subject of information individual client	has subject of information individual and / or family
has degree yes / no	has degree: no, mild, moderate, severe, complete	has degree the set of options from the selected judgment category
has potentiality actual	has potentiality actual	has potentiality actual
other characteristics do not apply	other characteristics do not apply	other characteristics do not apply
Conclusion: The focus for fear from NMDSN and ICNP are similar; ICF is different, it is too broad, although fear is one of the emotions falling under the b1522 code. This is not specific enough for nursing, where for all emotions a separate code would be required for documentation / statistical use. The judgment wording differs, but the meaning (concept level) is similar, indicating for all three that there is a problem situation. Subject of information is different for ICF (individual only) compared to the matching NMDSN and ICNP. Degree in NMDSN differs from the others, which use similar grading. Potentiality is similar for all three. Thus, this term cannot be mapped for individual care. It is possible to map for aggregate purposes, such as health statistics, or illustrating the diversity of patient populations, but only if it pertains to individuals and not to groups.		

Table 3. Dissection of 'Lack of motivation to co-operate in treatment and care'.

NMDSN item	**ICF concept**	**ICNP® concepts**
NMDSN	ICF ability	ICNP
has focus motivation has dimension cooperation in treatment and care	has focus motivation	has focus reason for action
has judgment lack of	has judgment impairment	has judgment insufficient or ineffective
has subject of information client	has subject of information individual client	has subject of information individual,
has degree yes / no	has degree: no, mild, moderate, severe, complete	has degree the set of options from the selected judgment categories insufficient / ineffective
has potentiality actual	has potentiality actual is perspective on fulfilling needs	has potentiality actual is perspective on understanding and explaining behaviour of the person.
Conclusion: This one does not match sufficiently, the focus, supported by the perspective on show different concepts. Also, additional attributes are supportive to reveal the meaning of the concepts better. These terms cannot be interchanged between NMDSN, ICF and ICNP®		

ual, family, or group. It is remarkable that many concepts from ICF and ICNP® can be exchanged easily. This works best for those concepts that need little detail, so for pain it is adequate, but it is not for a detailed pain assessment. Thus, if very specific details are important, such as in clinical documentation, further mapping and dissection are required. For the NMDSN it is not important.

2.3. Mapping

Because some of the 24 items from the NMDSN consist of multiple-choice items, the grand total of concepts used in the mapping and dissection is 39. It is assumed that for individual patient care information that is more detailed is necessary in comparison to aggregate purposes, like management information. The NMDSN is developed for aggregate purposes [7, 8]. Thirty-nine diagnostic concepts in the NMDSN are thus dissected via the characteristics of the ISO standard model for nursing diagnoses. This reveals the extent to which these terms can be interchanged in for example electronic messages, or aggregated for statistical purposes.

Table 4 shows the NMDSN items, the equivalents from ICF and ICNP®, and the extent to which they can be mapped.

Table 4. Level at which concepts from NMDSN, ICF and ICNP® Bèta 2 can be interchanged.

NMDSN item	Interchangeable for clinical purpose.	Interchangeable for aggregate purpose.
1. Problematic communication*	Reasonable individual care, not groups	Individual care only
2. Need for information, knowledge, or skills*	Only if there is no need for detail.	Individual care only
3. Fear*	No, ICF code is too broad.	Individual care only
4. Uncertain about the future*	Not at all	Not at all
5. Problems in contact*	Only if there is no need for detail. And only for individual care, not for groups.	Individual care only
6. No insight in health situation	Not at all	Not at all
7. Therapy / regimen	Not at all	Yes
8. Lack of motivation	Not at all	Not at all
9. Behavioural problems	Not at all	Not at all
10. Disorientation	Only for time, place and person	Yes
11. Thinking process / confusion	Not at all, more detail required	Yes
12. Restlessness	Not at all, more detail required	Yes
13. Pain	Yes	Yes
14. Problems with sleep/rest	Yes	Yes
15. Coping / stressful situations	Yes	Yes
16. Pressure ulcer (all 4 stages).	Not at all, more detail required	Yes
17. Impaired elimination	Not at all	Yes
18. Fever (high temperature)	Yes	Yes
19. Breathing problems	Yes, if the general concept is sufficient	Yes
20. Problems with food and fluids	Yes, if the general concept is sufficient	Yes
21. Self-care limitations	Yes, if the general concept is sufficient	Yes
22 Functional problems ADL 1 - walking / moving, 2 Prepare food, 3 – eating 4 - personal hygiene, 5 - Dress / undress, 6 - Change body position & 7 - Toileting	Yes, if the general concept is sufficient	Yes
23- High risk for complications, accidents, patient falls, infection and wound healing	Not at all	Not at all
23. High risk pressure ulcer	Not at all, more detail required	Yes
24. Life threat circulation, breathing and consciousness	Yes	Yes
25. Life threat elimination & temperature	Yes, if the general concept is sufficient	Yes

* indicates problems that can belong to either the patient or family, so can refer to group level.

3. Conclusion

It is possible to determine the semantic equivalence of terms from different terminologies that are used to describe similar concepts. The dissection reveals clearly what terms from NMDSN, ICF and ICNP® can easily be exchanged from one to the other without loss of meaning of the concepts for clinical and/or for aggregate purposes. Also, the conditions for interchange are made explicit, like for the four items for individual care only. For purposeful applications of the three terminologies under study, it is interesting to know that exchanging information, based on several of the terms can be done without information loss according to the dissection results. If aggregation from nursing documentation is required, and nurses in different settings use different terminologies, the use of mapping can help to bridge the terminological divide that often exists. This is consistent with approaches for the aggregation of nursing information [8].

Limitations however, exist in the origin of the NMDSN: it is largely based on the ICF's earlier version (then called ICIDH), which might cause some selection bias. Thus, additional mapping with other terminologies still needs to be done. Also, although the mapping between ICF and ICNP® has been established for the 39 example concepts, and the method does work, mapping of all other hundreds or thousands concepts from ICF and ICNP® would need similar work to be carried out. A reference terminology will eventually assist in preventing the mapping explosion due to too many combinations possible.

Dissections have revealed interesting findings about the usability of the ICF for nursing care, such as its unsuitability to describe nursing care for groups. This is an important requirement for nursing care and terminologies.

In addition, it is necessary to perform concept clarification for those concepts and terms from NMDSN, ICF and ICNP® that did not match or those that showed great differences in the dissection. It is especially important to pay attention to terms from the NMDSN that are semantically not consistent, i.e. it is not clear what concept they represent. Because we will face loss of information at aggregate level, this needs special attention to eliminate extra problems due to unclear descriptions.

Dissections based on the ISO model allow a detailed analysis of characteristics of terminologies, leading to discoveries of their usability. In this project, it was carried out for mapping between nursing diagnoses, which proves to be a valid option for use of the ISO standard. Given the adequacy of the ISO IS 18104 reference terminology model, to discover these characteristics from different terminologies, it can be considered as the 'gold standard' for scientifically sound and meaningful mappings between nursing classifications and terminologies.

However, the facilitation of mapping between nursing terminologies is only one of the suggested purposes of the ISO IS 18104 standard. The ISO IS 18104 should also be tested for its other purposes, like the examples presented [4, 5, 6]. The methodology to develop a terminology model is not new [2] and not exclusive for the nursing domain. It can be applied to several other health care terminologies to achieve a proper and meaningful exchange of information about patients and care. It is important that all disciplines that want to be part of the larger healthcare information exchange focus on harmonizing their terminologies in order to achieve the more unified reference health model.

In summary, we now have insight into how different nursing and healthcare terminologies relate to each other and how the ISO standard IS 18104 can be used to analyze and harmonize different nursing terminologies, and to support aggregation of nursing data via mapping. The ISO standard model and the required and optional attributes of nursing diagnoses provide a fit with terms from NMDSN, ICF and ICNP®. The IS 18104 does serve one particular purpose for which it is intended: it facilitates mapping between nursing terminologies.

Acknowledgement

This project was carried out under the mirror group on classifications and terminology of the Dutch normalization institute (NEN), under de acronym 'Nursys'. It was part of a larger project to translate the ICNP® Beta 2 into Dutch and test the CEN and ISO standard work for nursing. This was funded on a 50% basis by the National institute for ICT in Healthcare (NICTIZ).

References

[1] ISO TC 215 (2003). Health informatics - Integration of a reference terminology model for nursing. ISO/IS 18104.

[2] Rossi Mori A, Bernauer, Pakarinen V, Rector AL, De Vries Robbé P, Ceusters W, Hurlen P, Ogonowski A, Olesen H. (CEN / TC 251 / PT003), (1992). Models for Representation of Terminologies and Coding Systems in Medicine. In: Proceedings Seminar : "Opportunities for European and U.S. Cooperation in Standardization in Health Care Informatics". Geneva, CEN TC 251, 1992.

[3] CEN TC 251 (2000). Health informatics, systems of concepts to support nursing prENV 14032.

[4] Bakken, S., Warren, J.J., Lundberg, C., Casey, A., Correia, C., Konicek, D., & Zingo, C. (2002). An evaluation of the usefulness of two terminology models for integrating nursing diagnosis concepts into SNOMED Clinical Terms. International Journal of Medical Informatics; 68(1-3):71-77.

[5] Hwang JI, Cimino JJ, Bakken S. (2003). Integrating Nursing Diagnostic Concepts into the Medical Entities Dictionary Using the ISO Reference Terminology Model for Nursing Diagnosis. J Am Med Inform Assoc. 2003 Jul-Aug;10(4):382-8.

[6] Moss J, Coenen A, Mills ME. (2003). Evaluation of the draft international standard for a reference terminology model for nursing actions. J Biomed Inform.;36(4-5):271-8.

[7] Goossen WTF, Epping PJMM, Van den Heuvel WJA, Feuth T, Frederiks CMA, Hasman A. (2000). Development of the Nursing Minimum Data Set for the Netherlands (NMDSN): Identification of Categories and Items. Journal of Advanced Nursing, 31 (3), 536-547.

[8] Goossen WT, Epping PJ, Feuth T, van den Heuvel WJ, Hasman A, Dassen TW (2001). Using the nursing minimum data set for the Netherlands (NMDSN) to illustrate differences in patient populations and variations in nursing activities. Int J Nurs Stud;38(3):243-57.

[9] ICN, (2001). The International Classification for Nursing Practice (ICNP®) Beta 2. Geneva, ICN The International Council of Nurses.

[10] WHO (2001). International classification of functioning, disability and health: ICF. Geneva, World Health Organization.

[11] Coenen, A., (2003). Nursing Classifications "The International Classification for Nursing Practice (ICNP®) Programme: Advancing a Unifying Framework for Nursing". Online Journal of Issues in Nursing. Article published April 3, 2003 [Webdocuments http://nursingworld.org/ojin/tpc7/tpc7_8.htm accessed 2 October 2003].

[12] Hardiker, NR, (2001). A Logical Ontology for Nursing Interventions. Doctoral thesis University of Manchester Faculty of Science and Engineering.

[13] Hardiker, NR, Rector AL (2001). Structural Validation of Nursing Terminologies. Journal of the American Medical Informatics Association 8: (3) 212-221.

Contact information

William GOOSSEN PhD, RN
Acquest Research and Development,
Dorpsstraat 50 2396 HC Koudekerk aan den Rijn, the Netherlands,
T: +31715419594
F: +31715418202
@: williamtfgoossen@cs.com

A Web-based Support System for the Belgian Breast Cancer Screening Program

Eddy HUSSON[a], Michèle GUILLAUME[b] and Adelin ALBERT[c]
[a]*Informatique Médicale et Biostatistique, Université de Liège, Liège, Belgium*
[b]*Observatoire de la Santé de la Province de Luxembourg , Marloie, Belgium*
[c]*Informatique Médicale et Biostatistique, Université de Liège, Liège, Belgium*

Abstract. The Belgian Breast Cancer Screening program has been launched in 2002 according to the recommendations and quality assurance guidelines of the European Union. Women in the age range 50–69 years are invited to pass a mammography which is read by two independent radiologists. In case of discrepancy, a third reading is requested. Each reading is documented in detail. In the absence of a nationwide central support computer system, a novel Web-based computer system was designed and developed to support the program. The Web site is hosted on a Web server running Windows Server 2003 with Internet Information Server 6.0 and uses ASP technology from Microsoft. Patient data and readings results are entered from the Web site and are stored in an SQL Server database. The support system developed bears all the advantages of Internet-based facilities (e.g., low cost, remote data entry, flexibility, work comfort, ubiquitous access, user friendliness and advanced technology). Difficulties related to graphical data entry on Web pages were smartly resolved. A comprehensive algorithm for comparing mammography readings has been implemented in the system, enhancing the quality of the screening program. The application has been tested and implemented in the Province of Luxemburg, a widespread rural region particularly suited for Internet solutions in preventive medicine. More recently and with little efforts, the application was extended to the Province of Namur. The Web-based system provides management facilities, ubiquitous online statistics, and builds up a reservoir for official statistics and scientific research. As the application is concerned with sensitive medical data, special attention has been paid to provide a maximum of security. Administrative and medical personnel have expressed their total adherence to the system, while local health authorities have used it to justify their involvement in the screening program. Currently, the database for the Province of Luxemburg contains 25,321 women with a mean age of 59.5 ± 6.1 years (range: 50–70 years). The participation rate amounts 17.2%, about twice as much as in the other provinces. After the first mammography reading, 20.4% of the women were found to be positive, but this figure dropped to 10.2% after the second mammography reading. The overall disagreement rate between the first and second readings currently amounts 19.7%. It follows that a third reading is required in about 20% of the cases. Statistical analyses have shown that Cohen's Kappa agreement coefficients between radiologists range between 0.37 and 0.70. The application has been running for two years with success to the satisfaction of managerial and medical personnel as well as of provincial public health authorities.

The Minimum Medical Record for Practitioners on Duty (DMMG)

Didier LECLERCQ
CEO Professional Computing Solutions SA (PCSol),
Avenue Hanlet 5b, B-4802 Verviers, Belgium

Abstract. The Minimum Medical Record for Practitioners on Duty (DMMG) is a share and consultation platform containing all patient's essential medical data required in emergency cases. This prototype is now developed in the area of Verviers and in Eastern Belgium. The project is carried out by the *Meditel* non-profit-making organization and Professional Computing *Solutions* (PCSol).

The objective is to give to practitioners on duty, emergency services and mobile intervention teams a quick access to critical information about the patient, according to the duty lists. By this way, DMMG wants to improve the quality of care provided to the patients with respect to their rights. The aim is also to position the usual treating practitioner at the center of the healthcare process and to meet the new social challenges of emergency services.

The method used is a portal located on Internet with a high level of security. With the agreement of the patient, the treating practitioner transmits in a secure way to a central server all medical data that is considered as relevant in order to set up a minimum data file for the duty roles. Under the supervision of ASBL MEDITEL, access rights to the server are managed based on the active duty roles (GP and emergency practitioners).

DMMG data file is then available for all General Practitioners on duty, emergency practitioners and medical intervention vehicles (VIM). Remote reception of data (out of the hospital) is done on a laptop or PDA via GSM (GPRS) connection. In case of intervention, service on duty has access to DMMG. Every consultation or added information is transmitted to the Treating Practitioner in order to ensure healthcare continuity.

Results for the patient is the availability of reliable data about his health condition (responsibility of the patient for his health). He also avoids wasting time giving approximative medical explanations in difficult or emergency situations. The communication with the medical world is improved.

For the treating practitioner, DMMG optimizes medical data flows management and enables a prompt and precise diagnosis by others physicians even for patients at home. The physician is ensured of the healthcare continuity even during his absence. He stays in the middle of the healthcare process and he has a trust relationship with his patients and others colleagues.

Concerning the emergency services, DMMG allows an optimal management of this department by avoiding double examinations and speeding up patients handling.

Address : Professional Computing Solutions (PCSol)
Avenue Hanlet 5b
B-4802 Verviers, Belgium
Tel : +32 87 29 10 00 ; Fax : +32 87 22 39 66 ; info@pcsol.be
www.pcsol.be

The JaWS Project: Knowledge Engineering for Mobile Prevention Advisors

Dr Bart VIAENE[a], Dr Patrick VERCAMMEN[a] and Mr Vincent KEUNEN[b]
[a]*DEWE vzw*, [b]*MANEX sprl*

Abstract. *Objectives* : The recent legislation regarding "Well-being on the workplace" sealed a paradigm shift for nearly 100 Belgian external prevention services, leading to an important re-grouping movement – to 22 services at date – which has not yet found its final equilibrium. In the early nineties it became clear that new services requirements, multidisciplinary teams, higher quality standards – such as, recently, ISO 9001 – and the implementation of a medical "numerus fixus" at the universities would soon necessitate structural changes and the development of innovative instruments to meet future prevention needs.

The group IDEWE-IBEVE has played an active role in the genesis of the new legislation and the shift of traditional occupational health & safety prevention practices towards risk assessment, medical and environmental surveillance and psychosocial counselling at work, securing this revolution by the development of a modern software infrastructure to support its mobile prevention experts in a changing landscape.

Methods : The JaWS project is the largest effort in this novel support infrastructure. It centres around knowledge engineering: capturing and formalizing the wealth of expertise of a large multidisciplinary group of professionals, and applying it as building blocks in an auditing and reporting instrument suited to experts and novices alike.

The JaWS toolset is constructed to function as an automated refinery of expert knowledge, funnelling user-applied changes to a reviewing committee and redistributing useful improvements to all mobile prevention advisors.

Stochastic methods are applied to detect and research possible relationships between observations belonging to distinct prevention domain ontologies (industrial sectors, professions, hazards, health and safety problems, medical investigations…) and to guide preventive measures tackling surfacing trouble spots.

Results : Hundreds of mobile prevention advisors have been using JaWS for two years now, generating standardized and tailored advisory reports. A team of epidemiologists is developing feed-back procedures based on harvested observations, and ICT-experts are shaping the JaWS mobile application generator to make maximum use of future mobile computing platforms.

The JaWS project is gathering momentum, regularly integrating expansion modules into the auditing platform. JaWS symbolizes the fact that IDEWE is sinking its teeth in the delicate task of re-inventing its role in a changing industrial and legal landscape, on the never-ending quest of making prevention work.

A Medical Telematics Association in Brussels

Didier du BOULLAY, Lawrence CUVELIER,
Geneviève HANIQUE and Pierre LAMBRECHTS
The founding members of AbruMeT
Association Bruxelloise Médicale de Télématique

Abstract. *Objectives* : In the actual context of rapide changes in the health care environment, the need for efficient communications of medical data between the care providers became critical. Therefore, hospitals, general and specialised practitionners started dicussions throughout Belgium. These initiatives led to the constitution of non profit medical telematics associations (ASBL/VZW) which goals remain similar : the elaboration of medical networks after analysis of the needs and the implementation of exchange procedures. These associations will keep these medical networks under the responsibility and management of physicians who must assess the identification, authentication and certification of the potential users and guarantee the respect of the patients rights and privacy. The same discussions have started in Brussels. The goal is the implementation of a Brussels Medical Telematics Association. The name "ABruMeT" has been choosen to respect the utilisation of 3 languages : French (Association Bruxelloise Médicale de Télématique), Dutch (Associatie of Brusselse Medische Telematica), and English (Association of Brussels Medical Telematics).

Method : In 2003, delegates of general practitionners and hospitals started discussions. They defined what they want to do together and how, and summarised their willing in three issues. The first one is to get together, as far as possible, all the recognised associations of general pratitionners and all the hospitals situated in the Brussels area, and to avoid commercial or financial interests. Therefore, the ASBL/VZW formula was choosen. It implies the redaction of a juridical agreement, the implementation of a specific structure, and the respect of each members'sensibility. The second issue is the need for an active collaboration with the Telematics Commission of the Federal Ministry of Public Health. Finally, the third issue concerns the medodology which included three aspects detailled in the results: which informations do the health care providers need? Which are the technical needs and the available tools? How to work in accordance with the law defining the patients rights and privacy?

Results : The ASBL/VZW juridical agreement has been written, discussed and submitted to a lawyer. Some members participating to the working cessions of the Federal Telematics Commission, its projects and realisations have been immediatly integrated into the task list. The task list detailed the three aspects mentionned in the methodology. The needed informations have been described in the collaboration chart and include bilateral secured messages, protected access to a synthetised health care record for both partners, the bilateral alert concept and the access from outside to the inhospital patient record. Besides a minimal computer equipment and optimal securisation procedures for the data for both partners, we need secured channels and standardised codification and structure. Such standardisation is going on with the homologation of electronical health care records for general practitionners and the developpement of a common language : the KMEHR. Finally, the procedures must be implemented to permit the integration of the patients rights into a system with as final goal the quality and the continuity of care.

Digital Signature and Electronic Certificates in Health Care

Advice nr 2 of the Belgian Telematics Commission
"Telematics Standards in relation to the Health Sector"
www.health.fgov.be/telematics/cnst

1. Digital Signature and Electronic Certificates

1.1. The digital signature techniques (Note 1) and procedures offer more guarantees and advantages (e.g. in terms of integrity and authentication) than hand-written signatures. Digital signatures should therefore be recognised as valid signatures and their use should be - when appropriate - encouraged in the health care sector.

1.2. The provision of registration and certification services (Note 2) is an essential requirement for achieving the levels of trust, security and quality in electronic communication as demanded by the health care sector.

1.3. In order to get the 'best practice', compliance is recommended with international laws, standardised rules and agreements applicable to such services (cf. Directive 1999/93/EC of the European Parliament and of the Council of 13 December 1999 on a Community framework for electronic signatures, published in the Official Journal of the European Communities, 19.1.2000). Liaison will also be established with the mixed national committee "Information Society".

1.4. A distinction has to be made between identity certificates and attribute certificates. The assessment of the identity and of attributes can be executed by different registration authorities. Several certificates can be associated with one pair of keys. The owner of certificates should be able to use every certificate separately (Note 3).

[Note 1] In the Working Group Security a distinction has been made between an electronic signature and a digital signature. The term 'Electronic Signature' is used in the context of 'legal validity or evidential force' whatever the technique used to get an Electronic Signature (eg. a smartpen). By 'Digital Signature', the WG means the technique where hashing and asymmetric encryption are used.

[Note 2] The registration authority checks the credentials of the applicant to grant a certificate. The certification authority produces the certificates. Certification can be on-line or off-line. Examples of different certificate-types are : identity certificates, qualifications certificate, 'role within an organization'-certificate, mandate-certificate, for legal entities: relationship-certificate.

[Note 3] Anybody (including eg. health professionals) should be in the possibility to make a selective use of certificates if he wishes to do so in particular circumstances (without being obliged to show other qualification-certificates which are then not relevant).

1.5. By Belgian Law, the Chamber of Physicians (through its Provincial Councils) and the Chamber of Pharmacists are the responsible authorities for the registration and revocation of physicians and pharmacists. In Belgium, there should be an agreement on the choice of the organisation(s) maintaining a complete directory with appropriate identification data on health care professionals (Note 4) in order to assess e.g. their identity and professional qualifications (Note 5). The Ministry of Health and Social Affairs could undertake such an initiative together with other relevant organisations (eg. Chamber of Physicians/National Medical Council, Council of Pharmacists…) and in co-operation with the Third Party Payer (RIZIV-INAMI). Such platform could serve as national registration authority for the professional qualifications and as interface with certification service providers (i.e. private companies acting as Trusted Third Parties).

1.6. A framework should define the roles, the rights, the responsibilities and the obligations of the different actors involved in secure services implementing digital signatures (cf. liability issue).

1.7. Where digital signatures are going to be used, health care information flows and communication scenarios (with type and purpose of message, type of sender and receiver (Note 6), identity certification need, attribute certification need) should be identified.

1.8. A key pair used for digital signature purposes should never be used for other purposes.

1.9. Proof of identity should be stored as close as possible to the person as such. Private keys used for digital signatures can be stored on smart cards which are considered safe.

1.10. Access rights to resources should be kept close to the system and managed by the organisation responsible for the decision and/or implementation of access.

1.11. Multifunctionality should be promoted; i.e. it should be made possible of having several attribute-certificates linked with one single identity.

1.12. In the case a conflict of interest might (Note 7) (Note 8) arise from the different qualifications of a single person it is the responsibility of that person to use the right attribute-certificate(s) (the inclusion of a certificate should be a 'conscious'act: this is a non-technical issue). User applications should nevertheless follow procedures to warn, ask and incite, where appropriate, to include the 'right' certificates.

Note 4 By health care professionals is meant not only physicians (general practitioners or specialists) but also all other health care actors such as nurses, pharmacists, dentists, logopedists, dieticians,… and health care administrative personnel.

Note 5 A physical person can have several qualifications (corresponding with attribute-certificates) granted by different organisations or institutions (delivered by certification authorities).

Note 6 The communicationpartners can be either natural persons or artificial persons in private and public law or even machines (e.g. servers).

Note 7 E.g. clinican and/or medical adviser of an insurance company and/or industrial medical doctor and/or inspector.

Note 8 A Working Group member still believes that, in the case of conflict of interest (antagonistic qualifications) and in the interest of the patients, two identity certificates offer more guaranties than one identify certificate with two or more attribute certicifates. This is in contradiction with what the rest of the Working Group believes.

1.13. Attribute-certificates can – under certain circumstances – be used without identity-certificate or with pseudonyms.

1.14. Certificates should never be delivered behind one's back. Verification should be made possible. The person should be informed.

2. Trust Services

2.1. In the health care sector there is an absolute need for services from Trusted Third Parties (TTP). The roles of such trust service providers can be very diverse as they can offer services in various security domains such as Public Key Infrastructure (PKI) support (key management, smart card personalisation and distribution, directory services, etc.), anonymisation and pseudonymisation services (Privacy Enhancing Techniques, PET) and notary services (eg time and date stamping, proof of delivery).

2.2. Priorities for health care sector are the PKI services (to enable the implementation of digital signatures in health care) as well as anonymisation and pseudonymisation TTP (to enable the unlocking of data for eg medical research and management purposes).

2.3. Guidelines for such TTP services in health care should therefore be drafted.

References

[1] Directive 1999/93/EC of the European Parliament and of the Council of 13 December 1999 on a Community framework for electronic signatures.

[2] Belgisch Staatsblad - 17.03.2000 - Moniteur Belge Ministerie van Ambtenarenzaken - N2000 - 688 [C - 2000/02025], 12 Maart 2000 - Koninklijk besluit tot oprichting van een Nationale Gemengde Commissie.

[3] F. De Meyer, F. Allaert, G. De Moor, T. Fiers, Arguments en faveur de la reconnaissance de la valeur juridique de la signature électronique, Informatique et Santé, 1996 (8):23-35 - Springer-Verlag France.

[4] G. De Moor, F. De Meyer, Beveiligingsaspecten met betrekking tot elektronische medische gegevens, Tijdschrift voor Geneeskunde - Volume 53 - Nummer 5 - 1 maart 1997.

[5] Y. Poullet, R.J. Barcelo, Working Document based on the article: Health Telematics Networks: Reflections on Legislative and Contractural Models Providing Security Solutions, Centre de Recherches Informatiques et Droit (CRID), University of Namur.

[6] P. Van Eecke, Bewijsrecht en digitale handtekeningen: nieuwe perspectieven, To be published in "Belgische Vereniging van Bedrijfsjuristen", 1999.

[7] Digital Certificates, GlobalSign NV, Apr-99.

[8] Synthèse des décisions prises lors des réunions CARENET tenues les 1er, 15 juillet et 4 août 1999 concernant la certification des messages, en présence des représetants de l'INAMI, de la BCSS, du Ministère de la Santé publique et des organismes assureurs. Bruxelles, le 17 août 1999.

[9] Working Group "11-19" on Security Standards (www.11-19.org/security.html).

[10] Projet de loi n° 322 relatif à l'activité des prestataires de service de certification en vue de l'utilisation de signatures électroniques. La Chambre. 27/01/2000.
Wetsontwerp nr 322 betreffende de werking van de certificatiedienstverleners met het oog op het gebruik van elektronische handtekeningen. De Kamer. 27/01/2000.

Implementation Framework for Digital Signatures for Electronic Data Interchange in Healthcare

Georges DE MOOR[a], Ir. Brecht CLAERHOUT[b] and Ing. Filip DE MEYER[c]
[a]*Department Medical Informatics and Statistics, University Hospital Gent, Belgium*
[b]*Custodix NV, Merelbeke, Belgium*
[c]*RAMIT vzw, Merelbeke, Belgium*

Abstract. This paper aims to propose an action plan for the deployment of the use of digital signatures in Belgian healthcare.

This action plan is the result of a number of technical, legal and organisational requirements. It starts by establishing the functional components that are needed to set up a framework for the deployment of digital signatures. The main components should implement an infrastructure for:

- the creation of digital signatures;
- the verification of digital signatures;
- the certification of signature keys;
- the certification of attributes;
- the handling of revocation.

The tasks in the action plan are the logical consequence of all the functions that need to be addressed.

The objective of this report is to list what has to be done and how it can be done in the context of healthcare, rather to state who will perform the functions required.

Keywords. Digital signatures, Trusted Third Party, Registration Authorities, Certification Authorities, Public Key Infrastructure, Digital Certificates

1. Background and Rationale

As the storage and communication of data is becoming more and more digital, the need becomes clearer to consider the legal value of transactions and documents. For paper documents procedures have been established that attribute legal validity, and the procedures for the flow of these documents have been described (e.g. hand-written signatures). The present text describes the requirements for the provision of a trustworthy digital equivalent of this functionality. Rather than concentrating on 'confidentiality of content' issues or on privacy issues of the actors or citizens involved (encryption[1]), it focuses on mechanisms for the following properties:

- protection of the integrity of the document. This implies that no part of the document has been changed since the document was signed and that the document is complete;
- non repudiation of actions. This means that actions on documents, such as sending, receiving, or opening are attested and time-stamped;

[1] Although a remark on encryption functionality is made in Section 4.6.

- non repudiation of content by the signatory;
- the ability for a signer to sign in a certain capacity or role, which is a healthcare specific aspect.

In legislation the term 'electronic signature' is used to avoid the restriction of legislation by the state of technology at a given time. Currently, however, the only practical solution for electronic signatures is the use of digital signatures, i.e. electronic signatures based on the use of asymmetric encryption within the framework of a PKI (Public Key Infrastructure) that provides all the supportive functions necessary for deployment and use.

The use of electronic signatures is not specific to healthcare alone. This project therefore will draw upon resources from any domain involving technical solutions and choices. Nevertheless, the framework within which the signature and certification functions will be deployed is specific to healthcare. Technical and operational choices need to be adapted to the particular Belgian healthcare context.

The document has been drafted in English because of the technical nature of its terminology. It is a basic text to be used in a bilingual environment and it can be translated on demand.

2. Healthcare Flows (Certificates)

In addition to the creation of a PKI infrastructure that allows the use of digital signatures, it is important to establish what documents have to be signed and by whom.

The following non-exhaustive list contains documents that require a signature of a medical doctor (the English terms are translated from the Dutch terms used in Flanders):

✓ medical certificates for:
  - medical care provided (doctor or hospital receipts, tax receipts)
  - disability for work
  - school absence
  - social leave (parental leave, leave for illness of family member)
  - illness invoked for cancellation insurance
  - the inability to give informed consent (mental incompetence, e.g. dementia)
  - urgent medical assistance
  - death
  - birth

✓ treatment prescriptions:
  - medicines
  - physiotherapy

✓ refund applications:
  - medicines
  - orthotic appliances

✓ medical inspection documents:
  - accidents
  - insurance
  - recruitment
  - intoxication
  - assistance to third parties, integration allowance, income support
  - parking permit
  - social benefits
  - admission to a rest home or nursing home

✓ requests for specialist or hospital care and laboratory medicine:
  - radiology
  - clinical laboratory
  - pathological anatomy
  - referral
  - hospitalisation: admission, prolongation, discharge

✓ minimum clinical data set registration

Further categories of documents that require signatures include:

✓ docket for magnetic cards
✓ receipt for out-patient invoicing
✓ attestation for delivery by surgical truss-makers
✓ individual out-patient medication invoice
✓ collective hospitalisation invoice
✓ statement of out-patient invoices
✓ statement of normal out-patient rehabilitation services
✓ statement of rehabilitation oxygen therapy
✓ monthly statement of laboratory tests for out-patients
✓ statement of blood products and derivatives
✓ summary list of table of statements

3. Explanatory Part

3.1. Definitions

Non-repudiation
Definitions of non-repudiation may vary slightly, depending on the context. The definition adopted here is: "non-repudiation is a signer's inability to deny that he has signed the document"

PKI – Public Key Infrastructure
The set of hardware, software, people, policies and procedures needed to create, manage, store, distribute, and revoke Public Key Certificates (PKCs) based on public key cryptography.

CA – (Public Key) Certification Authority[2]
An authority trusted by one or more users to create and assign public key certificates.
The CA may create the user's keypair (private and public key).

It must be observed that the CA is responsible for all certificates during their entire lifetime, not just for assigning them. A CA can certify both end users and other CAs.

Root CA
The most trusted Certification Authority (CA), which is on top of a certification hierarchy. The Root CA has a self-signed certificate, which means that this entity has to be trusted by all members of that Public Key Infrastructure (PKI).

Subordinate CA
A Subordinate CA is a CA that has been certified by another CA.

[2] The terms 'Certification'/'Certificate'/'Certifying' Authority are all used in literature.

ACA – Attribute Certification Authority (also called AC Issuer)
An authority trusted by one or more users to create and sign Attribute Certificates (ACs). It is important to note that the ACA is responsible for the attribute certificates during their whole lifetime, not just for issuing them.

RA – Registration Authority
An entity charged with performing some of the administrative tasks necessary in the registration of subjects, such as confirming the subject's identity; validating that the subject is entitled to have the values requested in a Public Key Certificate (PKC), and verifying that the subject has possession of the private key associated with the public key requested for a PKC.

ARA – Attribute Registration Authority
The equivalent of a public key RA for attribute certificates, i.e. a supporting entity for the Attribute Certificate Authority (ACA) issuing Attribute Certificates (ACs).

PKC – Public Key Certificate
A data structure containing the public key of a person or organisation (CA or ACA) and some other information, which is digitally signed with the private key of the CA that issued it. The information contained in the Public Key Certificate (PKC) should be sufficient to uniquely link the certificate to a real person or organisation.

AC – Attribute Certificate
A data structure containing a set of attributes for a person or organisation and some other information, which has been signed digitally with the private key of the Attribute Certification Authority (ACA) that issued it. The information contained in the AC should be sufficient to uniquely link the certificate to a real person or organisation or to an existing Public Key Certificate (PKC).

Repository
A database service capable of storing information, such as certificates and Certificate Revocation Lists (CRLs), allowing unauthenticated information retrieval. Repositories include, but are not limited to, directory services.

Certificate Holder
An entity that is named as the subject of a valid certificate.

CRL – Certificate Revocation List
A CRL is a time stamped list identifying revoked certificates that is signed by a CA, ACA or CRL issuer and made freely available in a public repository.

DTS – Digital Time-stamping Service
A DTS issues time-stamps that associate a date and time with a digital document in a cryptographically strong way. The digital time-stamp can be used at a later date to prove that an electronic document existed at the time stated on its time-stamp.

3.2. An Introduction to Digital Signatures

This section gives a short overview of the technology behind the digital signature, and introduces the concepts of Public/Private key pair, Public Key Certificate (PKC) and Public Key Infrastructure (PKI).

3.2.1. Digital Signatures

Digital signatures are created and verified by means of cryptography, the branch of applied mathematics that deals with transforming messages into seemingly unintelligible forms and back again. For digital signatures two different keys are generally used: one for creating a digital signature or transforming data into a seemingly unintelligible form, and another key for verifying a digital signature or returning the data to its original form. Computer equipment and software using two such keys are often referred to as an "asymmetric cryptosystem".

The keys of an asymmetric cryptosystem for digital signatures are termed the 'private key', which is known only to the signer and is used to create the digital signature, and the 'public key', which is ordinarily more widely known and is used to verify the digital signature. A recipient must have the public key corresponding to the private key in order to be able to verify that a digital signature is the signer's. If a large number of people need to verify the signer's digital signatures, the public key must be distributed to all of them, perhaps by publication in an easily accessible on-line repository or directory.

Although the keys of the pair are mathematically related, it is computationally infeasible to derive one key from the other, if the asymmetric cryptosystem has been designed and implemented securely for digital signatures. Although many persons will know the public key of a given signer and use it to verify that signer's signatures, they cannot discover that signer's private key and use it to forge digital signatures.

The use of digital signatures comprises two processes, one performed by the signer and the other by the receiver of the digital signature:

- **Digital signature creation** is the process of computing a code derived from and unique to both the signed message and a given private key. For that code or digital signature to be secure, there must be at most only a negligible chance that the same digital signature could be created by any other message or private key.
- **Digital signature verification** is the process of checking the digital signature by reference to the original message and a public key, and thereby determining whether the digital signature was created for that same message using the private key that corresponds to the referenced public key.

A more fundamental process, termed a "hash function", is used in both creating and verifying a digital signature. A hash function creates in effect a digital freeze frame of the message, a code usually much smaller than the message but nevertheless unique to it. If the message changes, the hash result of the message will invariably be different. Hash functions enable the software for creating digital signatures to operate on smaller and predictable amounts of data, while still providing a strong evidentiary correlation to the original message content.

As illustrated in Figure 1, in order to sign a document or any other item of information, the signer first delimits precisely what is to be signed (the "message"). Then a hash function in the signer's software computes a hash result, a code unique to the message, called the message digest. The signer's software subsequently transforms the hash result into a digital signature by reference to the signer's private key. The resulting digital signature is thus unique to both the message and the private key used to create it.

Typically, a digital signature is attached to its message and stored or transmitted with its message. However, it may also be sent or stored as a separate data element, as long as it maintains a reliable association with its message. Since a digital signature is unique to its message, it is useless when completely dissociated from its message.

Verification of a digital signature, as illustrated in Figure 2, is accomplished by computing a new hash result of the original message by means of the same hash function used in creating the digital signature. Then the verifier checks whether the newly computed hash

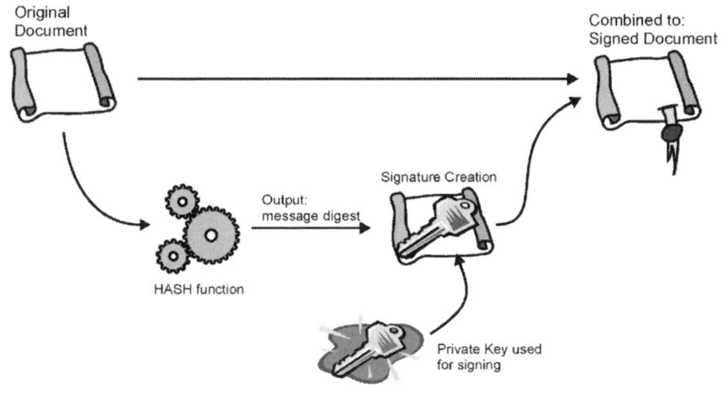

Figure 1. Digital signature creation.

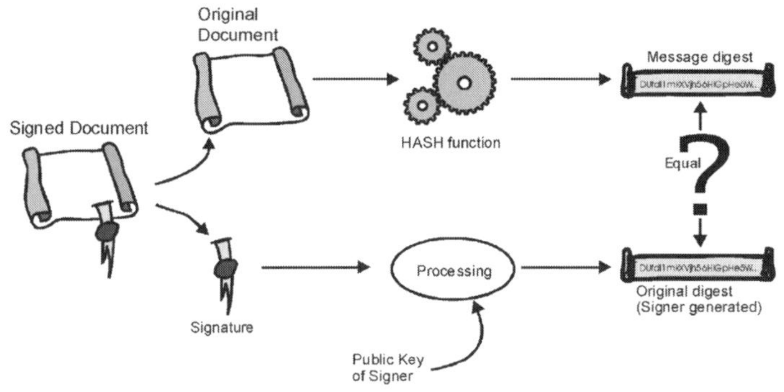

Figure 2. Digital signature verification.

result matches the original hash result calculated from the digital signature using the public key. If the hashes match, the digital signature is verified. Verification thus indicates (1) that the digital signature was created using the signer's private key, and (2) that the message has not been altered since it was signed.

Various asymmetric cryptosystems create and verify digital signatures using different mathematical formulas and procedures, but all share this overall operational concept.

The processes of creating a digital signature and verifying it achieve the essential effects a signature should have:

- **Signer authentication**
  If a public and private key pair is associated with a single identified signer, a digital signature by the private key effectively identifies the signer with the message. The digital signature cannot be forged by a person other than the proper signer, unless the latter loses control of the private key, such as by divulging it or by losing a computer-readable card and its associated personal identification number (PIN) or pass phrase.
- **Message authentication**
  The process of digitally signing also identifies the matter to be signed, typically with far greater certainty and precision than paper signatures. Verification also reveals any tampering with the message, since processing the hash results (one made at signing and another at verifying) discloses whether the message is the same as when signed.

The core algorithms used for digital signatures have undergone thorough peer review, and an extensive scientific and technical literature underlies them. Digital signatures have been accepted in several national and international standards developed in co-operation with and accepted by many corporations, banks, and government agencies. The likelihood of malfunction or a security problem in a digital signature cryptosystem designed and implemented as prescribed by the industry standards is extremely remote, and far smaller than the risk of undetected forgery or alteration on paper or of using other less secure electronic signature techniques.

3.2.2. Public Key Certificate (PKC)

To verify a digital signature, the verifier must obtain a public key and be ensured that it corresponds to the signer's private key. However, a public and private key pair has no intrinsic association with any person, as it is simply a pair of numbers.

In a transaction involving two parties the parties might succeed in bilaterally identifying each other with the key pair each party will use, but achieving such an identification is no small task, especially when the parties are geographically distant from each other, communicate over an open, insecure information network, are not natural persons but corporations or similarly artificial entities, and act through agents whose authority must be ascertained. Since reliably identifying a remote party involves considerable effort, establishing a remote party's digital signature capability especially for each of many transactions is utterly inefficient. Instead, a prospective digital signer will often wish to identify himself with a key pair and reuse that identification in multiple transactions over a period of time.

To that end, a prospective signer could issue a statement such as "Signatures verifiable by the following public key are mine". However, others doing business with the signer may well be unwilling to take the signer's own purported word for its identification with the key pair. Especially for electronic transactions made over information networks rather than face to face, a party would run a great risk of dealing with a phantom or an impostor, or of facing a disavowal of a digital signature by claiming it to be the work of an impostor. To assure that each party is indeed identified with a particular key pair, third parties trusted by both others must associate an identified person at one end of the transaction with the key pair creating the digital signature received at the other end, and vice versa. That trusted third party is generally termed a Certification Authority (CA).

To associate a key pair with a prospective signer, a Certification Authority issues a certificate in the form of an electronic record that sets forth a public key and states that the prospective signer (or "subscriber") identified in it holds the corresponding private key. Thus a certificate's principal function is to identify a key pair with a subscriber, so that a person verifying a digital signature by the public key listed in the certificate is ensured that the corresponding private key is held by the person listed in the certificate.

To assure the authenticity and inviolability of the certificate, the Certification Authority digitally signs it. The issuing Certification Authority's digital signature on the certificate can be verified using the public key listed in another certificate, and that other certificate can be verified by the public key listed in yet another certificate, and so on, until the person relying on the digital signature is adequately assured of its genuineness.

3.2.3. Attribute Certificate (AC)

The relationship between a real identity and a public key is not the only one that can be certified digitally in the way described above.

It may sometimes be necessary that a person be required to prove in the digital domain that he has certain characteristics, e.g. being a doctor. Certificates proving someone's characteristics or more specifically linking certain attributes to a person are called Attribute

Certificates (ACs). The issuers of these certificates are called Attribute Certificate Authorities (ACAs), by analogy with Certificate Authorities. The certifying techniques are the same as for PKCs, i.e. a fixed format message containing information on the certificate holder's attributes is signed by the issuing ACA.

The ACs themselves are linked to an identity (the certificate has to link its attributes uniquely and non-repudiably to a person or organisation) by listing the identity of the person directly in the certificate (preferred method) or by referring to the person's PKC.

3.2.4. Public Key Infrastructure (PKI)

Turning the theory of public key cryptography, and digital signatures in particular, into a useful, real-world system requires more than just the implementation of the core algorithm. A number of supporting operational elements need to be in place before public key cryptography can be used effectively. The supporting infrastructure is collectively known as Public Key Infrastructure, or PKI.

A PKI consists of a set of policies, procedures and services to support applications of public key cryptography. The operational issues of running a PKI include how keys should be managed, how users have their identities checked, and how a specific user's public key is made available to other users. Most PKIs have the following main constituents:

- a Security Policy;
- one or more Certificate Authorities (CAs) and possibly one or more Attribute Certificate Authorities (ACAs);
- one or more Registration Authorities (RA) and possibly one or more Attribute Registration Authorities (ARAs);
- one or more Repositories.

Security Policy

The security policy contains definitions of the actual operation of the PKI. The operation of each PKI component should be detailed here, as well as procedures for key generation, issuance, storage, and revocation. In effect the security policy is the framework for the PKI.

Certificate Authority (CA)

As explained above, a CA issues Public Key Certificates. It is responsible for the certificate during its complete lifetime (from issue date to expiration date).

Once issued, a certificate may prove to be unreliable sometime before expiration. For example, if the subscriber loses control of the private key, the certificate becomes unreliable, since digital signatures created by the lost private key would appear to be the subscriber's according to the certificate. In such situations, where the certificate has become unreliable, the certification authority may suspend (temporarily invalidate) or revoke (permanently invalidate) the certificate. Immediately upon suspending or revoking a certificate, the certification authority must publish notice of the revocation or suspension, or at least notify persons who inquire or who are known to have received a digital signature verifiable by reference to the unreliable certificate. The security policy of a PKI should therefore contain a revocation policy and describe the mechanism for revocation.

Several CAs can co-exist, either side by side or in a hierarchical structure. Apart from issuing end-user PKCs, CAs can also sign each other, stating that they accept certificates issued by another CA as equivalent to their own. The many topologies and systems of interaction that exist between CAs are beyond the scope of this introduction.

Attribute Certificate Authority (ACA)

The Attribute Certificate Authority's operation is completely equivalent to the CA's, but deals with attribute certificates only. CA and ACA functions are often combined into one entity.

Registration Authority (RA)
When a user applies to a CA for a digital certificate, the CA has to verify that the applicant truly is who he claims to be. In most PKIs the strictly administrative task of verifying one's identity in the real world is separated from the technical task of signing a certificate. The role of the Registration Authority is to provide this verification. A real-world analogy would be with a notary public. Certain legal contracts require the signing to be witnessed by a notary, who verifies the signer's identity. In a similar way the RA verifies the applicant's identity and passes the application on to the CA. The degree of rigour applied by the RA during the verification will affect the degree of trust in the digital certificate. Some PKIs actually use notaries to act as RAs – an applicant physically signs a form, witnessed and notarised by a notary, before their PKC is issued by the CAs.

Attribute Registration Authority (ARA)
Attribute Certificate Authorities accredit a person with a certain attribute (e.g. a role). Analogous to the RA/CA relationship, an Attribute Registration Authority (ARA) assists the ACA administratively. These ARAs should check whether an applicant is entitled to the requested Attribute Certificate.

Repository
A repository includes, but is not limited to, directory services. A directory service is the PKI equivalent to a telephone directory. A telephone directory is used to look up someone's telephone number, a directory service to look up someone's digital certificate. Apart from the digital certificates a repository can also list revoked certificates.

4. Proposed Solution

4.1. Problem Definition

The main objective of a scheme for digital signatures in Belgian healthcare is to allow a healthcare professional (HCP) to sign documents in his different roles in such a way that signer authentication, message integrity and non-repudiation are guaranteed.

For large-scale (nation-wide) deployment of the solution to be feasible, it should comply with global standards and, if possible, mature technology should be chosen for its implementation.

4.2. Healthcare PKI Architecture

4.2.1. Introduction

Healthcare professionals (HCPs) act flexibly in several capacities or roles. They can sign a single document in various capacities at the same time or they can sign multiple documents in different roles. This is the case for a general practitioner or a specialist who works part-time for an insurance company as a medical expert. When requesting medical information about a patient he must distinguish between his roles and clearly state this in his electronic communication.

When HCPs are acknowledged in their specific function by different organisations, multiple certifiers co-exist on a technical level. Typically, an HCP will be accredited by some co-ordinating organisations and by a number of local organisations.

A naive and unrealistic approach to this problem consists in providing a new Public Key Certificate (PKC) for each role an HCP takes up. This would result in an unmanageable system that is doomed to collapse when deployed on a nation-wide scale. To name but a

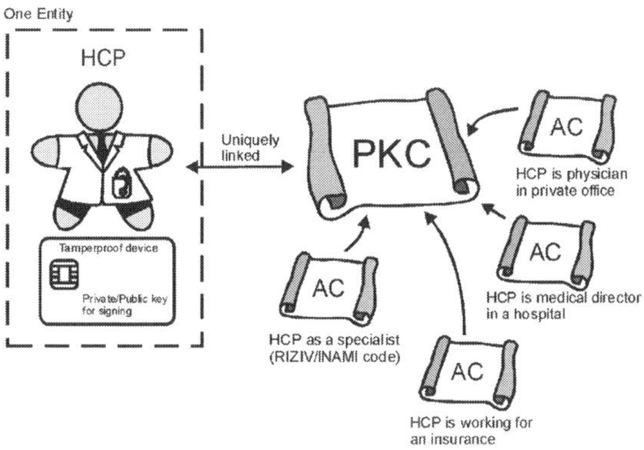

Figure 3. A healthcare practitioner and his certificates.

few drawbacks, a person would possess several private/public key pairs for his function as an HCP. This would undoubtedly create both logistic (key storage) and management problems. Signing in multiple capacities would be quite inconvenient (one document would be accompanied by multiple signatures).

This sort of solution is absolutely impractical. It is mentioned here only to illustrate the difficulties that are tackled by the PKI architecture further suggested in this document. Besides, such a solution does not correspond at all to the hand-written equivalent. When signing paper documents in different roles, one always uses the same (hand-written) signature. In such a case the capacity in which one signs is often listed next to the signature (as an attribute), e.g. 'CEO' when signing a contract in the role of company executive.

4.2.2. Architecture

Structure

The proposed solution avoids these problems by using one Public Key Certificate (PKC) per HCP and a set of Attribute Certificates (ACs). The PKC binds a public key to a person, thus identifying him within the digital domain (Figure 3). The attribute certificates (ACs) link a certain role (capacity, characteristic) to a person, or rather to his public key or his PKC.

In short, an HCP possesses a public/private keypair for signing all healthcare related documents (its use is not restricted to healthcare, see below). He will also possess a PKC that binds his public key to his identity. As the PKC should remain valid over a long period of time, it must not contain any information on the HCP's position in the healthcare system (often changing), but only information about his identity in order to bind his person uniquely to the digital key.

Next to the PKC, the HCP possesses a set of ACs that not only describes, but also proves his different roles in the medical system. These ACs range from nation-wide certificates (e.g. the right to practice as a doctor in Belgium) to local certificates (e.g. a certificate as a medical superintendent in a hospital).

For clarity's sake: ACs are separate entities. Some will be mutually exclusive, so that an HCP never signs in certain capacities at the same time, and thus never use the two ACs together, other ACs will be frequently used together.

Architecture and Health Authority Platform

The previous paragraphs show that different (local or national) accrediting organisations should be able to certify an HCP for a certain function. Such accreditation will be imple-

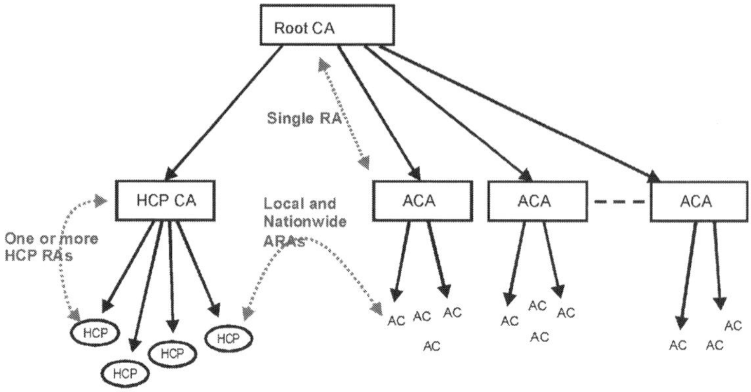

Figure 4. Proposed architecture of the Belgian healthcare PKI structure for digital signature.

mented as an Attribute Certificate (AC) linked to a PKC, which means that these organisations need to act as an ARA and/or an ACA. Forcing all the accrediting organisations to act as an ARA only would not only create an immense overhead for a centralised ACA, but it would also be illogical as certain roles are managed by the local organisation (e.g. a physician accredited as the head of a hospital department). It follows that all local organisations willing to accredit HCPs should be encouraged to implement an ACA. As this scheme provides for multiple certificate issuers, a policy should be determined for their interaction.

Next to the accrediting of HCPs a structure for binding them to a public key is required. In contrast to the ACA/ARA requirements, this is a centralised function.

The proposed architecture to implement these requirements is shown in Figure 4. It is a strictly hierarchical CA architecture (2 levels) with a single Root CA (Root CA being the top level CA, i.e. the third party everybody trusts in a strictly hierarchical PKI).

The top level CA issues only subordinate CA certificates, certifying two kinds of authorities: a HCP CA and several ACAs. The HCP CA issues one and only one PKC per healthcare practitioner, which certifies the unique link between a public key and a specific HCP. Because the HCP CA is a subordinate CA to the Root CA, extension to multiple[3] HCP CAs is possible with little or no impact on the entire structure (and implementation). It also allows merging with the Belgian initiative on the electronic ID card (see Section 4.5).

As explained above, the ACAs issue only Attribute Certificates (ACs), and no Public Key Certificates (PKCs). These ACAs represent the technical branch[4] of accrediting organisations that need to certify an HCP's function in the 'national' healthcare system (i.e. a function that has significance outside the scope of the organisation). These accrediting organisations (e.g. hospitals, third party payers, etc) should all be certified by the top level CA.

A major task in the proposed digital signature framework solution is that of registration (i.e. RA or ARA). There are three main different types of registration in the scheme as shown in Figure 4. First of all, one single RA should be responsible for the registration of new accrediting organisations in the healthcare digital signature scheme. There is no need (though it is possible) to divide this task among multiple RA organisations, as it is expected to be a small task once initial introduction of the network is completed.

---

[3] It is expected that one single HCP CA will suffice for the Belgian healthcare system.

[4] Which can be contracted out.

A second registration task is the support of the HCP CA (or maybe multiple HCP CAs at a later stage). The HCP RA (or RAs) are responsible for verifying the identity of HCPs so that a public key can be uniquely bound to an identity.

Finally, the ARAs takes up the administrative part of accrediting HCPs with certain healthcare roles. It is clear that many ARAs will co-exist, some dealing with nation-wide accreditation (e.g. the RIZIV/INAMI could issue a certificate that services performed by a certain HCP are covered by the social security system), others with regional/local accreditation (e.g. certifying someone as a medical superintendent in a hospital). As explained above, because of technical limitations not all institutions will have a proper ACA, but several organisations can share this technical functionality, while remaining responsible for their own registration.

The main functions in this architecture (Root CA and corresponding RA, HCP CA and HCP RA, some national ACAs and ARAs) should be implemented by a Health Authority Platform[5]. This Health Authority Platform could consist of the major healthcare related bodies in Belgium, like for example the Ministry of Health, the RIZIV/INAMI, the professional associations (chamber of physicians, chamber of pharmacists, etc), the future federal database of healthcare practitioners, etc. The exact allocation of functions within this platform is however outside the scope of this document. It is clear that several institutions can and will fulfil different roles, e.g. the Department of Health could act as HCP RA, RA and as ARA.

The proposed architecture meets all functionality requirements while remaining relatively simple. Allowing multiple top level CAs, islands of trust, using deep levels of certification, all are possibilities that make the PKI architecture even more flexible. But many PKI initiatives have failed because of their urge to use all available technical features. The architecture proposed here is not only adequate and scalable, but, if implemented properly, it allows expansion to any complex architecture in a later phase (if at all necessary). It is our experience that the setting up of such an architecture on a national scale is a strong enough challenge already.

Key Management

Key Storage

The secrecy of one's private key is the principle underlying the digital signature system. Once a person's private key is compromised, an attacker can impersonate that person in such a way that no distinction whatsoever can be made between documents signed by the genuine certificate holder and the impostor.

We therefore advise that private key storage be only allowed on appropriate tamperproof storage devices such as smartcards or security tokens. Disk storage of sensitive private keys should be prohibited.

The reasons for this are quite obvious. Everyone having access to a computer where a private key is stored, can copy it. Even if the key is encrypted, an attacker can take it home and try to break the encryption. Usually users use weak protection mechanisms to protect such things as keys stored on a disk (simple passwords), which makes matters worse. People also tend to copy their private key on each system they use it on, thus the key gets spread, increasing the security risk. Tamperproof secure devices do not have these disadvantages. Private keys cannot be extracted from such cryptographic devices, thus they can never be backed-up (copied and spread). These devices do the cryptographic calculations internally, only presenting the result of the calculation to the outside world, not the private key. Furthermore, protection against compromise of the private key after loss or theft of the

[5] Or contracted out, under their responsibility.

device exists. Access is protected with a password, and the device disables itself after a few unsuccessful access attempts.

Key Generation
Ideally the signer generates his keypair and sends the public key to the CA to obtain his Public Key Certificate (after verification of his true identity and right to certification). In this way the private key never leaves the signer (subscriber), who maintains full control over the operation and is therefore completely certain that his key did not get compromised during the certification process.

In the Belgian healthcare situation, however, this certification method is hardly feasible. We therefore advise that keypairs be generated and issued by the HCP CA. *Appropriate technical (tamperproof devices) and legal measures should prevent access to the generated private key by the HCP CA.*

Certificate Management

Public Key Certificate Distribution
To verify a signature on a document, first and foremost the PKC of the signer is needed. Common practice is to list these certificates online at central points (directory service).

The proposal for the Belgian healthcare system provides for only one HCP CA issuing PKCs (possibly expanded to multiple HCP CAs on the same level, if needed), allowing easy centralisation of such a directory service. Such a function could be contracted out, preferably to organisations already having an operational infrastructure.

The two-layer structure of the proposed PKI, makes verifying the genuineness of the public key quite simple. Only a HCP CA certificate and the Root CA certificate are needed, and both can be stored locally on the end-users' systems.

Thus the chain of certificates needed to verify a signature is in this case restricted to the signer's PKC, an HCP CA certificate, and a single Root CA certificate. Therefore it is recommended that in this situation documents be always accompanied by the relevant PKC to facilitate signature verification.

Attribute Certificate and ACA Certificate Distribution
As the attribute certificates listing the HCP role are always included in the signed document (see 4.3), no additional distribution mechanism is needed. The ACA certificates needed to verify the ACs could also be included in the document (see below). If this is not the case, the verifier will have to obtain them first. The ACs provided should therefore list the location of the ACA certificate repository.

Certificate Revocation
A major aspect of certificate management is certificate revocation. A CA or an ACA is responsible for a certificate from the day it is issued to the day it expires. If for some reason the certificate were to be considered invalid (e.g. private key compromise), it should be possible to make this public.

There are two main methods for managing revoked certificates. One is to distribute lists (Certificate Revocation Lists, CRLs) with revoked certificates on a regular basis. Checking revocation of a certificate takes place with a locally stored copy of the issued list (i.e. an off-line certificate revocation mechanism). The other is to check on-line for revocation each time a certificate has to be verified (e.g. by the Online Certificate Status Protocol, OCSP).

One of the problems with the first system is time granularity. Until the next list update, a revoked certificate may still be operational if the verifying party cannot get the latest information by any other means. There are several procedures in the revocation management protocols to overcome the most obvious problems with CRLs, such as growth of the CRL

(Delta-CRLs, Partitioned CRLs), simultaneous update of all local CRL lists (Overissued-CRLs), ...

On-line revocation check has the disadvantage of creating large amounts of traffic when a large number of certificates need to be checked, and thus creating problems of network connectivity. This method is generally used in environments where real-time certificate verification is essential for correct operation, e.g. online payment.

In a first phase, an off-line revocation system using certificate revocation lists is a sufficient means of revocation for the Belgian healthcare system. CRLs contain the unique serial numbers of the certificates that were revoked by a CA or ACA. These CRLs are typically distributed centrally by the CA/ACA in charge.

The healthcare information system has three entities issuing certificates. The Root CA issues subordinate CA certificates, the HCP CA issues HCP PKCs, and the ACAs issue the Attribute Certificates. As each CA/ACA is responsible for the certificates it issues, they should be responsible for their CRL distribution. This means that if they are unable to organise a CRL distribution point (there will be many small ACAs), they should contract it out. Typically, Health Authority Platform members could organise large distribution points. To manage this cluster of CRL distribution points we advise that inclusion of the location of the CRL in the certificates is mandatory. Each certificate issued should list an URL with the location of the CRL that could list this certificate.

An important part of the revocation policy is that of determining the CRL expiration period ("when should the local CRL copy be updated?"). The AC CRLs would typically have a much higher expiration rate than the PKC CRLs.

Key and Certificate Lifetime

Keys (i.e. corresponding certificates) and ACs should not be valid indefinitely. An important aspect of operational and certificate management is deciding on the lifetime of the certificates. Several aspects should be taken into account when drawing up the related policies: legal aspects (validity of signed documents), logistic aspects (signature keys should be valid for a long period, i.e. several years), management aspects for key replacement, etc.

Different certificates will clearly need different lifetimes. HCP PKCs will obviously need long validity periods, some ACs could have short periods of validity (e.g. for roles representing a temporary function).

4.3. Operational Procedures

4.3.1. Creating and Verifying Documents

This section describes the common operational procedure in the proposed digital signature infrastructure. First of all, the method of creating a signature in a certain healthcare capacity is described, and then necessary additional services to create a fully functional, reliable and trustworthy digital signature system are explained.

When an HCP wants to sign a document his digital signature application should prompt him to indicate in which capacity he wants to sign. Depending on the capacities in which the HCP wants to sign, different ACs corresponding to those capacities are attached to the original document by the software (Figure 5). It would be good practice to include the corresponding ACA certificates for the ACs to simplify the work of the verifier. This composed document should then be signed by the HCP's private signature key.

The signature now proves that the HCP himself has signed the composed document and that it has not been altered since. This not only means that the content of the medical document was approved by the signing HCP, but also that he signed in the capacity as listed by the ACs, because the attached ACs could not possibly have been tampered with unless the HCP's private key was compromised.

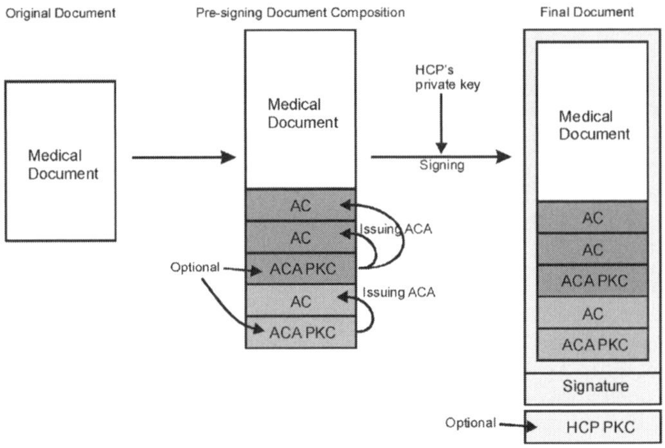

Figure 5. Construction of a signed document.

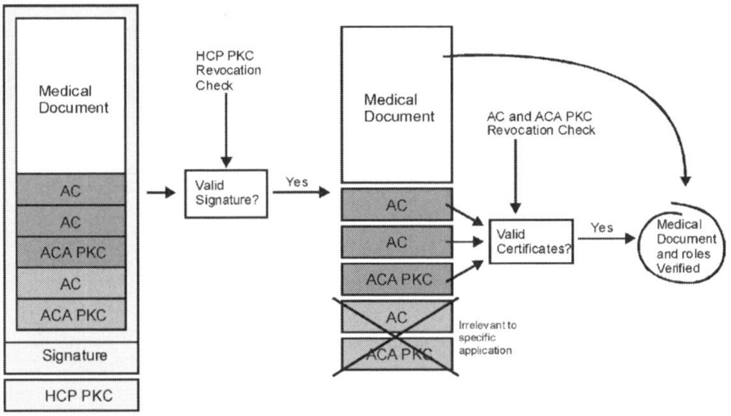

Figure 6. Verification of a document.

The final document can then be stored or forwarded. It is recommended to attach the corresponding signer's PKC to the final document, as this facilitates the verifier's work (no directory search). As explained above, the two-level hierarchy requires only the signer's PKC to verify one's trustworthiness (considering the fact that each entity has a local copy of the root CA certificate and HCP CA certificates).

Supplying all the necessary certificates for verification is often called a "push" mechanism, whereas a "pull" mechanism forces the verifier to search actively for the necessary certificates in repositories. Due to the nature of this application, the use of a "push" mechanism should be considered and could even be made mandatory.

The verification steps are straightforward (Figure 6). First of all, the origin and the integrity of the document should be checked by verifying the signature. If the signature verifies positively, then the composed document proves to be unaltered and effectively signed by the holder of the public key used for verification.

Depending on the application, certain attributes of the signer need to be checked. To do so, the application should search for the necessary ACs attached to the verified document.

If found, the validity of the ACs should be checked. The AC's origin can be verified by using the issuing ACA certificate while the latter can be checked with the root CA certificate. If the ACA certificates are not included in the signed message, they will have to be fetched first. Their location should be listed in the ACs. Again, possible expiration or revocation of each certificate has to be checked.

4.3.2. Long Time Storage, Time-Stamping

The described system of document verification presents one serious problem. After a key or an AC expires, anything that was signed with that key, or that contained the AC, will no longer be considered valid. If a signed document must remain valid after the signature key or ACs expire, the document should be time-stamped by a Digital Time-stamping Service (DTS)[6]. A DTS issues a time-stamp that associates a date and time with a digital document in a cryptographically strong way. A time-stamp proves that the digital document existed at the time stated. It is the digital equivalent of a notary service.

If the signature key or an AC expires or gets revoked after document time stamping, the document can still be verified as valid. Time stamping should be performed by a trusted party. A policy and protocol should be devised to avoid time stamping of documents that contain revoked ACs or that are signed with a revoked key.

For the sake of confidentiality, the contents of the document need not be revealed to the DTS. The author can compute a message digest of the document using a secure hash function and then send the message digest to the DTS, which returns a digital time-stamp consisting of the message digest, the date and time it was received, and the digital signature of the DTS.

To allow revocation checks of the ACs and key used for signing the document, the author could send both the message digest and a copy of all certificates used to the DTS. The DTS could then check all certificates, and include them with the message digest in the digital time-stamp. A time-stamp of a document can be considered genuine if the hash verifies and all certificates (or unique references to them) used are included in the time-stamp itself. Another method could be splitting the DTS into an administrative body, which is permitted to see the complete document for certificate verification, and a technical body, which performs the actual time stamping.

The above explanation is merely an illustration of the time-stamping principle. In reality DTSs take additional technical measures to guarantee the trustworthiness of their services.

Digital Receipts

In some scenarios an HCP needs confirmation that the document he sent has been received by the other party or proof that he has actually filed his document on time. In other words, the HCP wants a receipt for his document. A receipt proves that a transaction between two entities has taken place.

A receipt could be a message composed of a unique reference to the original document (a message digest), the date of reception (optionally a third party timestamp), and possibly some extra information (e.g. the original sender). This message should then be signed by the receiver and handed over to the sending HCP. If needed, the receipt could also include ACs in the same way as the signed document. Technically speaking, a receipt is nothing more than another signed document.

Non-repudiation

True non-repudiation is difficult to implement. An HCP can sign a document and subsequently claim that he did not. Consider the following example: first the HCP signs a docu-

[6] Also called a Digital Time-stamping Authority (DTA).

ment in the usual way. Later he denies that he himself signed the mentioned document and he claims that his private key was compromised before the signature date of the examined document. Although the same problem arises with the CA and ACAs, they can be considered trusted in the proposed scheme (policy). Use of tamperproof devices (smartcards) and DTS (time-stamping services) can, however, limit the effect of this type of cheating. There are other methods to reduce this risk, but their description is beyond the scope of the present document.

The above should be considered a technical remark that is made to avoid any arguments. Nevertheless, digital signatures can be regarded as non-repudiable within the administrative context of a given set of a strict (legally binding) policy and rules, and considered as more secure than their paper counterparts.

4.4. Normative References

The architecture proposed in this document can only be implemented successfully on a realistic time-scale and if it is based on existing standards.

The infrastructure and methods listed above have been proposed with widely accepted standards (or drafts) in mind, a non-exhaustive list of which follows:

- ✓ ISO/TS 17090-1:2002
  Health informatics – Public key infrastructure
  Part 1: Framework and overview
- ✓ ISO/TS 17090-2:2002
  Health informatics – Public key infrastructure
  Part 2: Certificate profile
- ✓ ISO/TS 17090-3:2002
  Health informatics – Public key infrastructure
  Part 3: Policy management of certification
- ✓ Various IETF/RFCs regarding X.509 PKIX, including but not limited to:
  - RFC3280: Internet X.509 Public Key Infrastructure Certificate and CRL Profile
  - RFC2527: Internet X.509 Public Key Infrastructure Certificate Policy and certification Practices Framework
  - RFC3261: Internet X.509 Public Key Infrastructure Time-Stamp Protocol (TSP)
  - RFC3281: An Internet Attribute Certificate Profile for Authorisation
- ✓ Various IETF/RFCs regarding S/MIME, including but not limited to:
  - RFC 3369: Cryptographic Message Syntax
  - RFC 2633: S/MIME Version 3 Message Specification

4.5. Healthcare PKI Architecture and the National Identity Card

The decoupling of identity and healthcare role in the proposed digital signature infrastructure allows a high degree of flexibility in its implementation. The private/public keypair used for signing and verifying a signature is not linked at all to the healthcare function. In other words, the PKC of the HCP does not contain any information on the fact that he is actually an HCP, it merely links a public key to a real-world identity. This means that the PKC should not necessarily be issued by a governing healthcare body. As long as the end-user PKC CA (HCP CA) is trusted nation-wide and acceptable for all HCPs and healthcare organisations, it can be used for the healthcare digital signature framework.

These conditions are perfectly met by the initiative taken by the Belgian government to introduce the electronic national identity card (BELPIC – BELgian electronic Personal Identity Card). This e-ID card will give every citizen the possibility to authenticate himself and to create signatures in the digital world (i.e. it will contain keypairs and certificates).

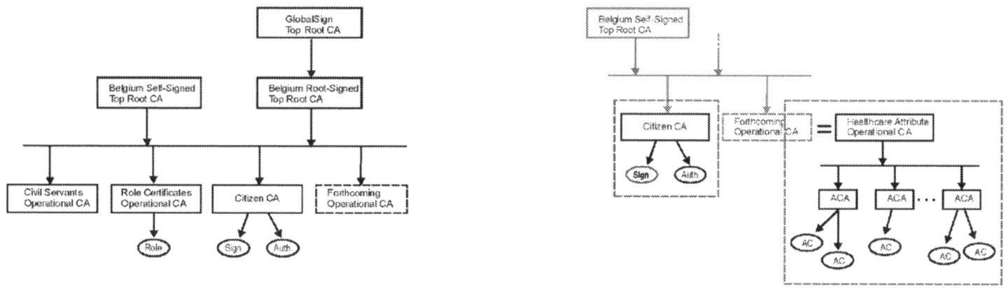

Figure 7. (a) Structure of Belgian e-ID CA hierarchy (b) possible merging of healthcare digital signature platform.

Figure 7a shows the structure of the Belgian CA hierarchy (as it is known to the authors today). As all functions needed for a digital signature (as required in healthcare) are present, healthcare practitioners could use their e-ID card for this function. The implementation of Certification Authorities within the healthcare digital signature framework could then be limited to a 'Healthcare Attribute CA' and its subordinate ACAs, as illustrated in Figure 7b.

Basically, the Root CA of the stand-alone architecture (Figure 4) becomes subordinate CA to the 'Belgian Top Root CA' and the 'HCP CA' is replaced by the 'Belgian Citizen CA'.

Integration of the healthcare digital signature framework in the Belgian PKI structure would not only simplify implementation and reduce costs, but also promote maintainability, user-friendliness, and general acceptance of e-government services.

The work on the national ID card has already reached the point where these cards are being actively tested. However, nation-wide distribution of the eventual e-ID card will take more than one year. It is now being studied how accelerated distribution among specific target groups such as HCPs could be encouraged in order to allow early use of infrastructures relying on the digital signature architecture. If this is not possible, it might be necessary to look for a temporary hybrid solution, before merging the national e-ID card with the digital signature infrastructure for healthcare purposes.

4.6. Merging to an Encryption Framework

The following notes on expanding the architecture for digital signatures to encryption may be beyond the scope of this document in the strict sense, but they are relevant to the issues discussed here.

Basically, what is needed for encryption is a new keypair (reasons are given below), the distribution of encryption keys (i.e. public key certificates containing the keys) and the means for revocation. As with the signature keys, encryption keys can be certified by a Certificate Authority (CA) to bind them to an identity (to ensure that encryption is done for the correct person).

Separate keys are commonly used for signing and encrypting[7] for a number of reasons. First of all, the nature of signature keys and of encryption keys is quite different. Encryption keys should be backed up to ensure the recovery of data that has been encrypted by them. Digital signature keys on the other hand must never be backed up, because they need to stay in the users' control to ensure non-repudiation.

[7] And for authentication.

Secondly there is the issue of security. The more frequently a key is used, the greater the chance that it will be compromised: a key may get lost, breaking a key becomes more profitable if more information is secured by it, more ciphertext[8] allows more effective cryptanalysis, etc. Therefore, it is advisable to use keys with a short lifetime, but this would logically be very inconvenient for signature keys. Thus one would want a shorter lifetime for encryption keys and a longer lifetime for signature keys, which implies different key pairs. Furthermore, if data is both signed and encrypted with the same public key pair, subtle weaknesses might be introduced that render the data vulnerable.

Because signature keys need a longer lifetime, a greater key length (stronger security) can be chosen without having to worry about performance, because this is usually not an issue for signatures (whereas it often is for encryption). Also, as far as implementation is concerned, there is a reason for splitting the keys. Not all digital signature algorithms are fit to be used for encryption. RSA can be used for both, DSA is a signature-only algorithm.

Because of the shorter lifetime for encryption keys, key management becomes more complex and time-consuming for CAs. To reduce the workload, users could take upon themselves some of the responsibilities by using the digital signature infrastructure. They could certify their own encryption keys, binding the public encryption key to their identity with their digital signature.

5. Action Plan

This document has proposed a solution for the introduction of digital signatures in Belgian healthcare. In order to deploy this framework the following action plan is proposed.

5.1. Consensus on the Proposed Model and Action Plan

The proposed PKI architecture, digital signature and action plan should be discussed and fine-tuned where necessary. Several decisions should be made before proceeding further (e.g. the interface with the BELPIC initiative).

It may be necessary to take into account information that is not currently available but still relevant to choices made in this document.

5.2. Establishment of a Health Authority Platform

Section 4.2.2 introduced the concept of a Health Authority Platform. This is the collection of healthcare bodies that will implement the different PKI authority functions (Registration Authorities, Certificate Authorities and Attribute Authorities). Once the model and the action plan approved, the different tasks within the proposed architecture must be assigned to the members of the Health Authority Platform.

5.3. Healthcare Domain Specifications

After allocation of the different responsibilities, the details specific for the healthcare domain should be elaborated. This includes:

- formatting Healthcare Roles in Attribute Certificates. Although at this point the transcription of all possible roles into attributes need not be determined, a global framework should be defined, to make gradual extension (new roles) of the attributes possible.

---

[8] Encryption generates a far greater amount of cipher text than digital signatures.

- healthcare specific elements of the operational procedure and dataflows should be defined (e.g. when Digital Time-stamping Services or receipts are needed).

5.4. Legal and Financial Studies

Important financial aspects may have to be considered. Existing legislation may have to be fine-tuned to ensure a robust legal and regulatory framework for healthcare. Operational procedures should be matched with present legislation. Topics such as duration of long time storage, non-repudiation and revocation policies should be dealt with.

5.5. Technical Specifications for RFP

At that point all elementary[9] aspects of the architecture, security policy, operational procedures (including protocols for signing, attaching ACs, creating timestamps, requesting and receiving receipts, interoperability guidelines, etc.) and workflows should be defined. This work should result in several detailed documents to be used as specifications for a Request For Proposal (RFP).

5.6. Launching a Tendering Procedure

Once the specifications are set, the tendering procedure can be launched.

5.7. Pilot Implementation

A pilot should be used to evaluate the implementation of the framework and allow for small changes to be made after review by end-users.

5.8. Deployment

After a successful test phase, nation-wide deployment should be planned. Care must be taken to allow a smooth transition to a uniform digital signature system. If the healthcare digital signature platform relies on the BELPIC initiative, the deployment of both systems will have to be synchronised.

6. The ISO PKI Technical Specification

6.1. Introduction

On 15 October 2002, ISO (International Standardisation Organisation) released the first edition of a technical specification of the way in which PKIs can be used to provide security services in general and digital signatures services in particular in healthcare. It describes the common technical, operational and policy requirements that need to be met for PKI to be used in the protection of the exchange of healthcare information. This Technical Specification is to be revised after three years and will then be turned into a full International Standard.

The Technical Specification comprises three documents:

---

[9] 'elementary' means that e.g. some details of the security policy can be left open for the RFPs.

1. Framework and overview: ISO/TS 17090-1 defines the basic concepts of a healthcare public key infrastructure (PKI) and provides a scheme of interoperability requirements for a PKI to be able to secure communication of health information.
2. Certificate Profile: ISO/TS 17090-2 provides healthcare-specific profiles of digital certificates based on the International Standard X.509 and the profile of this specified in IETF/RFC 2459 for different types of certificates.
3. Policy Management of certification authority: ISO/TS 17090-3 deals with management issues involved in implementing and operating a healthcare PKI. It defines a structure and the minimum requirements for certificate policies (CPs) and a structure for associated certification practice statements.

6.2. Relevance of this Document to the Belgian Situation

Rather than an international standard, the document itself is currently a technical specification intended as a guideline. This indicates that reaching a consensus on all aspects involved in setting up and operating a PKI is a difficult process. Nevertheless, the specification itself draws upon a number of established de facto and de jure standards that have been implemented into standard applications, e.g. Internet browsers, e-mail packages, etc.

The specification should therefore serve as a guideline for working out the specific tasks resulting from this project. The terminology list may also be of use to the wider community of different specialists involved.

The context of the document takes in more than just signatures, and only those parts that are relevant to the signatures issue are to be considered. Section 3 on management issues, in particular, is to be taken into account when setting up and operating a Belgian PKI healthcare solution.

According to the ISO PKI specification for healthcare, a healthcare PKI has to meet the following objectives to be effective in securing the communication of personal health information:

- reliable and secure binding of unique and distinguished names to individuals and organisations that participate in the electronic exchange of personal health information;
- reliable and secure binding of professional roles in healthcare to individuals and organizations;
- reliable binding of attributes to individuals and organisations.

These objectives shall be accomplished in a manner that maintains the trust of all who rely upon the integrity and confidentiality of the healthcare PKI.

7. Abbreviations

AC	Attribute Certificate
ACA	Attribute Certification Authority
ARA	Attribute Registration Authority
BELPIC	BELgian electronic Personal Identity Card
CA	Certification Authority
CRL	Certificate Revocation List
DSA	Digital Signature Algorithm
DTA	Digital Time-stamping Authority
DTS	Digital Time-stamping Service
HCP	HealthCare Professional/Practitioner
HCP CA	HealthCare Professional Certification Authority

HCP RA	HealthCare Professional Registration Authority
ISO TC215	International Standard Technical Committee on Health Informatics
OCSP	Online Certificate Status Protocol
PKI	Public Key Infrastructure
RA	Registration Authority
RFP	Request For Proposal
RSA	Rivest-Shamir-Adelman
URL	Universal Resource Locator

References

[1] Directive 1999/93/EC of the European Parliament and of the Council of 13 December 1999 on a Community framework for electronic signatures.

[2] Loi fixant certaines règles relatives au cadre juridique pour les signatures éléctroniques et les services de certification – Wet houdende vaststelling van bepaalde regels in verband met het juridisch kader voor elektronische handtekeningen en certificatiediensten.9.2.2001. Moniteur Belge/Belgisch Staatsblad 29.9.2001, pp. 33070-33078.

[3] Projet de loi n° 322 relatif à l'activité des prestataires de service de certification en vue de l'utilisation de signatures électroniques. La Chambre. 27/01/2000.- Wetsontwerp nr 322 betreffende de werking van de certificatiedienstverleners met het oog op het gebruik van elektronische handtekeningen. De Kamer. 27/01/2000.

[4] Arrêté royal déterminant les données relatives aux fournitures à tarifier que les offices de tarification doivent transmettre aux organismes assureurs. – Koninklijk besluit tot vaststelling van de gegevens inzake te tariferen verstrekkingen die de tariferingsdiensten aan de verzekeringsinstellingen moeten overmaken. 15.6.2001. Moniteur Belge/Belgisch Staatsblad 27.2.2001, pp. 25430-25446.

[5] Arrêté royal relatif à l'extension du réseau de la sécurité sociale à certains services publics et institutions publiques des Communautés et des Régions, en application de l'article 18 de la loi du 15 janvier 1990 relative à l'institution et à l'organisation d'une Banque-carrefour de la sécurité sociale. 16.1.2002. Moniteur Belge 6.2.2002, pp. 4072-4076.

[6] Arrêté royal prolongeant l'application de l'arrêté royal du 16 octobre 1998 portant des dispositions relatives à la signature électronique, qui s'applique à la sécurité sociale, en application de l'article 38 de la loi du 26 juillet 1996 portant modernisation de la sécurité sociale et assurant la viabilité des régimes légaux des pensions. 13.7.2000. Moniteur Belge 4.10.2000, pp. 33723-33724.

[7] De gecoördineerde wet betreffende de verplichte verzekering voor geneeskundige verzorging, 14.7.1994.

[8] Arrêté royal relative à la force probante des données enregistrées, traitées, reproduites ou communiqués par les dispensateurs de soins et les organismes assureurs, 27 Avril 1999, Moniteur Belge 15.5.1999, pp. 16799-16801.

[9] Projet de loi portant création de la banque de données fédérale des professionnels des soins de santé.

[10] Telecommunications Security; Electronic signature standardization report, ETSI.

[11] ETSI ES 201 733, Electronic Signature Formats, ETSI.

[12] Consensus visant à la compatibilité des systèmes de signatures numériques, AGORA.

[13] Recommendation No R (97) 5 of the committee of ministers to member states on the protection of medical data.

[14] Projet de Loi portent création de la banque de données fédérale des professionnels des soins de santé, Doc502022/006, 25.11.2002.

Corresponding author:

Prof. Dr. G. De Moor
Ramit vzw
Verlorenbroodstraat 120, bus14
B – 9820 MERELBEKE, BELGIUM
Tel: +32 9 240 34 36 - Fax: +32 9 240 34 39 - Email: georges.demoor@ugent.be

Recommendations Regarding National Development of Standardized Electronic Health Care Messages

Advice nr 4 of the Belgian Telematics Commission
"Telematics Standards in relation to the Health Sector"
www.health.fgov.be/telematics/cnst

1. Recommendation 1: XML

The use of the XML (eXtensible Markup Language) format is recommended as a syntax for health care messaging implementation.

Advantages of XML are its widespread industry acceptance, almost total support for XML throughout the world and global availability of an ever-increasing number of tools such as editors and browsers. In addition, it is demonstrated that XML has a number of benefits for storage or exchange of medical record information.

2. Recommendation 2: Generic Message Structure

The generic message structure defines a simple, minimal and practical framework for the exchange of clinical data.

2.1. Overview

- A message is composed of a header (including the communication parties – sender and recipients, and the date and time of the creation of the message) and one or more exchanged documents related to one or more patients.
- A document is a container for an amount of information that is linked to one and only one single patient.
- A document contains one or more transactions related to the patient concerned by the document.
- A transaction is defined as the information generated about a patient by a single author (who is responsible of the accurracy of the information) at one point of time (the creation date and time).
  A transaction is commonly linked to a contact of the related patient within the health care system or an interaction, when the patient is not present, between a health care practitioner and the record of the patient.
  The information contained by a transaction encapsulates a cohort of clinical findings (or data entries) organized in items and/or collections.

A transaction does not contain other transactions.
Each transaction relates to a single transaction type (or name).

- An item is an elemental unit of data entry and is the smallest unit of information which remains meaningful when considered alone.
Each item relates to a single item type (or name) and has a content (or value).
The content of an item can be atomic (one single element) or compound (multiple elements).
The elements of an item can be a wide range of data types including text strings, numeric values, dates, files or reference to external stored files.
An item content can then accommodate any textual, numerical, quantity, time-related, coded (referring to a given coding scheme) or multi-media data type.
- A collection contains groups of data entries : it is a recursive structure for aggregation of additional collections, items or a mixture of the two.
Each collection relates to a single collection type (or name).
The collection structure allows contained item(s) and other collection(s) to be hierarchically organized and grouped under common data subject.

2.2. Detailed and Formal Description

The message and the message elements have the following minimal structure :

Message

➢ Message = Header + Document(s)

A message is composed of an header and one or more exchanged documents.

Message Header

➢ Header = [ID + Date + Time + Sender + Recipient(s) + Version/Level] + Services

The message header contains identification elements and services elements.

Identification elements are
- unique message identifier (ID),
- creation date and time,
- identification elements of communication parties – sender and recipient(s),
- version *(see recommendation 8)* and level *(see recommendation 3)* of the standard to which the message complies.

Service elements are
- request for acknowledgement,
- indication of urgency,
- references to other messages.

Document

➢ Document = [ID + Patient] + Transaction(s)

A document contains identification elements and one or more transaction elements.

Identification elements are
- unique document identifier (ID),
- patient identification element.

Transaction

- Transaction = [ID + Date + Time + Author + Agents + Type] + Item(s) + Collection(s)

A transaction contains identification elements and at least one collection or item.

Identification elements are
- unique transaction identifier (ID),
- creation date and time,
- author,
- one or more other related agents (validator,requester,provider) attributes (identification, date and time),
- type of transaction (coded).

Collection

- Collection = [ID + Type] + Item(s) + Collection(s)

A collection contains identification elements and at least one collection or item.

Identification elements are
- unique collection identifier (ID),
- type of collection (coded).

Item

- Item = [ID + Type] + Content

An item contains identification elements and a content (made of elements).

Identification elements are
- unique item identifier (ID),
- type of item (coded).

3. Recommendation 3: Standardization Levels

Four standardization levels are defined to allow a phased approach of the complexity of the messages implemented using the generic message structure.

3.1. Overview

The level A implements message, message header, document, transaction types, the file item type *(the content of the item is a file)* and the free item type *(the content of the item is a user-defined XML structure)*.

The level B implements collection types in addition to level A.

The level C implements other item types in addition to level B.

The level D implements coded item content in addition to level C.

Basic data types will be implemented while required.

3.2. Level A: Normalized Transaction Type

A message of level A contains transactions with one single file or free item.
Collection and other item types are not used.

- Transaction = [ID + Date+Time + Author + Agents + Type] + Item
- Item = [ID + (TypeFile | TypeFree)] + [File | Free]

3.3. Level B: Normalized Collection Type

A message of level B contains transactions with collections of file and/or free items. Collection types are used. Other item types are not used.

- Transaction = [ID + Date+Time + Author + Agents + Type] + Collection(s)
- Collection = [ID + Type] + Item(s) + Collection(s)
- Item = [ID + (TypeFile | TypeFree)] + [File | Free]

3.4. Level C : Normalized Item Type

Same as level B plus the use of other item types without coded item contents.
Same as generic message structure but coded item contents are not used.

- Transaction = [ID + Date + Time + Author + Agents + Type] + Item(s) + Collection(s)
- Collection = [ID + Type] + Item(s) + Collection(s)
- Item = [ID + Type] + Uncoded content

3.5. Level D : Normalized Item Content

Same as level C plus the use of coded item contents.
Same as generic message structure.

- Transaction = [ID + Date + Time + Author + Agents + Type] + Item(s) + Collection(s)
- Collection = [ID + Type] + Item(s) + Collection(s)
- Item = [ID + Type] + Coded content

4. Recommendation 4: Priority List for Implementation

The working group recommends the following priority list for implementation :

<u>Transaction types</u>

- Contact report
- Admission notification
- Discharge notification
- Death notification
- Admission letter
- Provisional discharge letter
- Discharge letter
- Laboratory test request
- Laboratory result
- Procedure request
- Procedure result
- Drug prescription
- Note
- Alert
- RCM/MKG
- RIM/MVG

- RPM/MPG
- Epidemiological survey

Item types

- Free item : the content of the item is a user-defined XML structure
- File item : the content of the item is a file
- Drug and drug therapy item
- Laboratory test and result item
- Clinical coded item

Basic data types

- Patient (including person identification and demographic data)
- Healthcare party (including person or institution identification and address representation)
- Code (with reference to a given coding scheme)
- Moment (date and time representation)
- Number (real, integer)
- Text (string and set of string)
- Boolean (logical data)
- File (embedded file or reference to external file)

Necessary collection, other item and basic data types will be implemented while required.

5. Recommendation 5: Creation and Maintenance of a National XML Templates Repository Server and a National Terminology Server

It is recommended that the generic message structure and necessary related elements should be implemented in the form of XML templates (DTD – document type definitions or Schema) using English terms.

The resulting templates, together with help documents for users, should be freely available on a national templates public repository web server.

The English terms of the templates should be translated and explained in national Belgian languages and these informations should be freely available on a national terminology public web server.

An permanent expert team for maintenance of the results and users assistance should be available.

6. Recommendation 6: Standard Coding Systems – Creation and Maintenance of a National Multilingual Coding Systems Server

Standard coding systems should be recommended.

The corresponding code lists, with the texts (in English and national Belgian languages) describing the code definitions, should be freely available, together with help documents for users, through a national multilingual coding systems public web server.

An expert team for maintenance of the results and users assistance should be available.

7. Recommendation 7: Existing International Standards

As for the current recommendation, the working group will consider CEN (Comité Européen de Normalisation – European Committee for Standardization) 13606 pre-norm

(Electronic healthcare communication) and GEHR (Good European Health Record) european model, together with national initiatives, namely Prorec conceptual model based on CEN 12265 pre-norm and the KMEHR (Kindly Marked-Up Electonic Health Care Record) project results, for further recommendations and developments about clinical health care exchange messages.

The working group acknowledges HL7 as a widely used international exchange standard for deployment within health care institutions. The reuse of HL7 messages, in particular administrative 'admission – discharge – transfer' (ADT) and orders messages, is recommended whenever appropriated.

8. Recommendation 8: Further Actions

The working group will validate a concrete XML *(recommendation 1)* implementation of the generic message structure *(recommendation 2)* and the proposed priority list of types *(recommendation 4)*.

The working group will consider in the future an enlarged list of transaction, collection, item and data types.

It is also proposed to enrich the generic message structure elements with attributes and modifiers fields.

As the generic message structure will evolve, a simple linear version scheme will be proposed having the following characteristics : a new version will be based on the previous version and each version will be uniquely identified with a systematic revision indentifier.

To allow secure and efficient data communication in complex contexts and environments, distribution rules have to be formalized and implemented.

References

Publications

[1] Considerations for a Memorandum of understanding on Intensifying the collaboration between CEN/TC 251 and HL7 (CEN/TC 251 doc no N99-106).
[2] Harmonising CEN and HL7 work, Some issues for discussion, CEN/TC 251, chairman (CEN/TC 251 doc no N00-003) 2000-01-30.
[3] Health Informatics, Electronic Healthcare Record Communication, Part 4 Messages for the Exchange of Record Information CEN/TC 251 PT029.
[4] Health Informatics, Electronic Healthcare Record Communication, Part 3 Distribution Rules CEN/TC 251 PT028.
[5] HL7 Standard version 2.3, 1997, Health Level Seven publication.
[6] HL7 Version 2.3 and Progress Toward HL7 version 3.0, M.J. Shafarman.
[7] Projet KMEHR : Rapport final, version 1.0, October 99.
[8] Carenet : objectives, functionalities, planning.
[9] Long-term storage of electronic healthcare information in XML format, Hans Peterson, The Park project, 01-01-2000.

Internet sites

CEN model	http://www.centc251.org
HL7	http://www.mcis.duke.edu/standards/HL7/hl7.htm
GEHR	http://www.gehr.org
KMEHR project	http://www.users.skynet.be/mb/kmehr.htm
PROREC model	http://www.users.skynet.be/mb/kmehr/kmehr4.htm
XML	http://www.w3.org/XML
XML implementation of PT29	http://www.clinical-info.co.uk/xmlepr.htm

Long Term Preservation of Hospital Patients Records

Advice nr 7 of the Belgian Telematics Commission
"Telematics Standards in relation to the Health Sector"*
www.health.fgov.be/telematics/cnst

The « Archives » working group of the Commission « Norms for Telematics in the healthcare sector » (in short « Commission Norms ») examined how to preserve patients records for the long term (electronic, photographic or paper records) in the hospital sector.

Contents of the patient record as well as of the medical record, objects of the present recommendation, have been defined by Royal Decree on 3 May 1999. Minimal general conditions have been established to which the medical record, as described in article 15 of the law on hospitals, coordinated on 7 August 1987, has to answer (Moniteur Belge, 30-07-1999).

The Royal Decree on 3 May 1999 indicates that the medical record has to be preserved in the hospital at least during 30 years. It does not mention any delay for the nursing record.

Given real logistic problems of storage that such 30 years delay induces for hospitals, the working group studied an adaptation proposal to make to this Royal Decree. Attention was focused on the double aim linked to patient record preservation :

- ✓ To assure continuity and coherence of care in the follow-up of the patient, from womb to tomb (birth to death) and
- ✓ To guarantee long term quality and availability of relevant data abstracted from patients records for epidemiologic studies and scientific research purposes.

Accounting and administrative documents are not concerned by the present recommendation.

*
* *

Upon reserve of further considerations in relation to hospital integration in telematics networks, and contingent to the role that the patient could play in the preservation of his records, the Commission "Norms for Telematics" approved the following recommendations:

1. Documents that make up patient records should all have a date and a validation author.
2. Documents storage should use techniques that prevent data falsification.
3. The Commission "Norms for Telematics" recommends to be in line with the legal prescription delay of the Civil Code (article 2262 bis § 2 of the Civil Code) and, therefore, to preserve **whole** patients records during at least 20 years since the last contact (encounter) of a "major" patient (18 year) with the institution, or after 18 year for a patient of younger age (article 2252 of the Civil Code: prescription does not run against minors in age).

   The last contact is defined as the discharge date of a hospitalized inpatient or the date of the last visit in ambulatory care (outpatient visit, including in emergency service, for technical examination, for treatment, or as day case) spontaneous or planned for the patient in a hospital.

4. Beyond the legal prescription delay of 20 years, **synthetic** patients records have to be preserved. These records should contain **at least** hospital inpatients discharge letters, outpatients visits reports, pathology reports and surgery protocols.
   The selection of the last problem list of the patient as well as the follow up of evolutions specific to some pathologies (diagnoses) is recommended.
   Except if a motivated conservation note has been ratified by the chief of staff physician, other documents **can** be destroyed (among which let's mention radiological images, electrocardiograms and electroencephalograms, nursing and paramedical records, and drugs prescriptions).
5. Preservation of patients records is under the liability of the hospital chief of staff-physician who will look in particular after security, validity, exhaustivity, confidentiality and availability of stored documents to be assured. The hospital archiving organisation might include storage outside the hospital. Documents preservation can be enthrusted to specialised firms in respect to article 16 of the law of 8 December 2002 on the "protection of private life in relation to personal character data processing".°
   As a consequence, it is suggested to modify the wording of the Royal Decree of 3 May 1999, so that "the medical record has to be preserved in the hospital" becomes "the medical record should be preserved **by** the hospital …". The localization of stored documents outside of the hospital should be available inside the hospital.
6. Documents that make up patients records might, in general, be electronic in nature (electronic computerized patients records), photographic (images, microfilms) or in paper. Conversion of paper documents in electronic or photographic documents and of photographic documents in electronic documents should use techniques that guarantee integrity of content and authenticity of the conversion result. Supports of unique rewriting ("write-once") are recommended, being electronic (for example CD) or photographic (for example microfilms), for the long term preservation of documents.
7. Possibilities to store patients records in the general archives of the Kingdom of Belgium should be examined.

Endnotes

* The Belgian Commission approved this text in plenary meeting on 18 June 2002.

° Law of 8 December 1992 on the protection of private life in relation to personal character data processing : Article 16 (partim) : « When data processing is enthrusted to a subcontractor, the person liable for the processing, or his proxy in Belgium, should … Upon advice of the Commission for the protection of private life, the King might dictate appropriate norms in matters of informatics security for all or some categories of processing.

Francis H. Roger France et al. (Eds.)
IOS Press, 2004

Coordination of Medical and Hospital Information

Advice nr 8 of the Belgian Telematics Commission
"Telematics Standards in relation to the Health Sector"*
www.health.fgov.be/telematics/cnst

Given

- ✓ the key role of the patient record, made at least of the medical record and of the nursing record;
- ✓ the quantity and the value of patient information generated by medical, nursing, paramedical, pharmaceutical, social, logistical and financial activities;
- ✓ the need to ensure quality and optimal data processing for the support, analysis and evaluation of all facets of a hospital work;
- ✓ the obligation to respect patient rights, private life and professional secrecy protection by high level security measures when any of these sensitive data is processed;
- ✓ the growing importance of communication or of these data sharing inside and outside the hospital;
- ✓ the unavoidable use of informatics and telematics for the production, the process, the exploitation, the valorization and archiving of these data, and
- ✓ the official agreement of physicians "specialists in health data management":

the "Hospital" working group of the Commission "Norms for Telematics in Healthcare" finds that the management of information, informatics and telematics should be structured in the hospital.

*

* *

In answer to this structuring need, the Commission recommends to create a "coordination function for medical and hospital information" in each hospital.

This function would be obtained by :

- ✓ the setting up of a **global "business" plan** in order to develop and to exploit information as well as informatics and telematics resources in the hospital, and
- ✓ to appoint a **multidisciplinary coordination group** mandated to approve the "business" plan, its evaluation and its updated versions.

The Commission "Norms for Telematics" feels preferable not to define a fixed model for the internal organisation, each institution being free to set up this function in relation to its needs and capacities.

However, the Commission recommends to include at least in the multidisciplinary coordination group, directly, or by delegation, the manager, the director, the chief of staff-physician, the chairman of the medical council, the head of the nursing department, of the medical imaging department, of the laboratory of clinical biology, persons in charge of pharmacy, and in charge of informatics department. This group will also include physicians with the title of specialist in health data management.

Appointments in the coordination group will be submitted to the approval of the manager.

*

* *

The "business" plan will include an **agenda** of actions and an **evaluation** procedure for results. It will plan **regular updates** at least annual.

The "business" plan will at least take into account :

- ✓ The coordination of the integrated and secure setting up of the **electronic patient record** in accordance, among others, of the Royal Decree of 3 May 1999 that specifies "minimal general conditions to which the medical record (as described in article 15 of the law on hospitals, coordinated on 7 August 1987) should correspond".
- ✓ The distribution of **liabilities** for the validity and quality of clinical and administrative data available in the hospital.
- ✓ The management of **communication** and of the patient electronic record data sharing with every authorized health care professional, in particular the physician in charge of the patient.
- ✓ The organisation of the needed data gathering and verification for establishing the **minimal clinical summary** (MCS) and the minimal nursing summary (MNS), their transfer on electronic device to the Ministry of Public Health in the required delays, and the interpretation of feedbacks.
- ✓ The analysis of clinical and administrative data available in the hospital in order to monitor management, to evaluate internally activities, and to proceed to scientific research.
- ✓ The setting up of a plan for **security** procedures, i.a. for access rights control, quality, preservation and communication of data that make the electronic patient record.

Endnote

* The Belgian Commission approved this text in plenary meeting on 15 October 2002.

Subject Index

Author Index